BUSHCRAFT
FIRST AID

BUSHCRAFT
FIRST AID

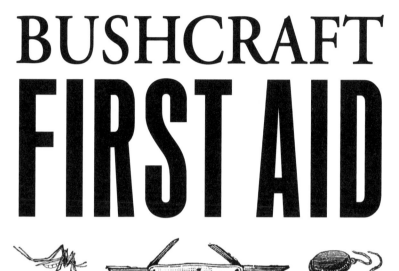

A Field Guide to
WILDERNESS
EMERGENCY CARE

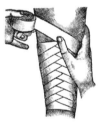

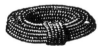

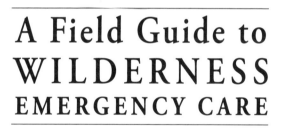

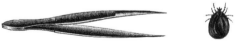

DAVE CANTERBURY

New York Times Bestselling Author of *Bushcraft 101*

& JASON A. HUNT, PhD

ADAMS MEDIA
New York   London   Toronto   Sydney   New Delhi

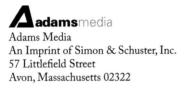

Adams Media
An Imprint of Simon & Schuster, Inc.
57 Littlefield Street
Avon, Massachusetts 02322

Copyright © 2017 by Simon & Schuster, Inc.

First Adams Media trade paperback edition JUNE 2017

ADAMS MEDIA and colophon are trademarks of Simon and Schuster.

For information about special discounts for bulk purchases, please contact Simon & Schuster Special Sales at 1-866-506-1949 or business@simonandschuster.com.

The Simon & Schuster Speakers Bureau can bring authors to your live event. For more information or to book an event contact the Simon & Schuster Speakers Bureau at 1-866-248-3049 or visit our website at www.simonspeakers.com.

Interior design by Colleen Cunningham

Interior illustrations by Eric Andrews

Insert-image credits listed at the end of this book

Manufactured in the United States of America

12 2021

Library of Congress Cataloging-in-Publication Data has been applied for.

ISBN 978-1-5072-0234-0
ISBN 978-1-5072-0235-7 (ebook)

DEDICATION

Dave: I would like to dedicate this book to my grandson Jax Conley. Being autistic and nonverbal, he may never have the opportunity to understand the words written in this book; however, it is my hope that this book will prepare others for the task of self-reliance and also aid in their ability to work within a group aiding and/or searching for others. Many autistic children by nature do not understand the dangers of life, like wandering off alone, or realizing, "If I walk into the lake I will drown." But like these children, we are all unaware of many dangers until we have been educated on how to avoid them or to deal with them if the need arises. Consider this a gift that hopefully will educate those who can comprehend these words from Jax and me to the future generations of outdoorsmen and outdoorswomen.

Jason: I dedicate this book to my wife, Robyn, and my children, Ethan, Sydnee, Lindsay, and Daniel, all of whom have allowed me to pursue that which God has laid on my heart to accomplish, regardless of how difficult or harebrained the tasks may have seemed at the time. I hope that as you each hold this book over the years to come that it serves as reminder of the promises of God and His goodness to our family and that by His grace, we have already overcome the world. Never lose heart, and follow your dreams; work hard and all you set your hand to shall be blessed. I love you all.

CONTENTS

CHAPTER 3: THE EMERGENCY SCENE 45

CHAPTER 4: TREATMENT OF BLEEDING AND WOUNDS 73

CHAPTER 14: INSECT AND ANIMAL BITES   181

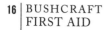

ACKNOWLEDGMENTS

Dave: I acknowledge with this fourth volume in the Bushcraft series all those who have taught before me. There are countless people through recent times who have inspired me and taught me invaluable lessons in both life and wilderness living. In no particular order these great men include Mors Kochanski, Steven Watts, David Wescott, Horace Kephart, Hyatt Verrill, Daniel Beard, Bernard Mason, George Washington Sears, and Ellsworth Jaeger. Men who have taught us not only through the written word but also by example that there is no true replacement for actual dirt time, experimental archaeology, and just plain grit to learn a valuable skill. I thank all of you for the contributions before mine and it is my honor to add to the volumes of outdoor guides that lead people to become more self-reliant.

Jason: I would like to acknowledge the emergency services community of which I am honored to be a small part. As a volunteer firefighter, first responder, and search team member I have been witness to hard work, sacrifice, and a sense of honor not often realized by those outside of this community. I would like to acknowledge specifically those who have had a direct hand in my training, without which this book would not have come to pass. William Rearden, chief of Kentucky River Fire & Rescue, has led by example over his twenty-plus years in the fire service. He has been the glue that has held the department together through adversity over the years, and without his leadership the people of Henry County, Kentucky, would have lost much-needed fire protection and rescue services. Mike Buresh, retired captain of

Bluegrass Search & Rescue, whose guidance in search theory, tactics, and leadership has served me well in life beyond the scope of search and rescue. And finally, Michael Payton and Connie Miller, without whose sacrifices my career in Emergency Medical Services would not have begun. Michael Payton, chief paramedic of West Lincoln EMS in Hustonville, Kentucky, passed away in the line of duty in 1998 and it was in his honor that a memorial scholarship was set up by his mother, Connie. I was selected as a recipient of the Michael Payton Memorial Emergency Services Scholarship Fund in 2011 and this gift, given in honor of a fallen brother in EMS, leader in his community, and son of a grieving mother, allowed me to begin my training toward becoming an EMT-B and later an EMS instructor, WEMT, and wilderness emergency care instructor trainer. I am grateful for leaders such as these and others around the world who serve without recognition; may God continually bless your service to your communities, departments, and families.

— Introduction —

WHAT IS WILDERNESS FIRST AID?

This book is for people who want to develop bushcraft skills so they can survive and thrive outdoors. One of the most important of these skills involves treating injuries and illnesses in the wild. Given that you probably won't be carrying a full line of splints, bandages, and medicines in your kit, you'll want to be able to use what's on hand to help deal with the problem. Knowing the basics of wilderness first aid can prepare you to be the first line of defense in an emergency.

Wilderness first aid (WFA) refers to the help you give someone who's been injured or becomes sick. It's not (and we can't stress this enough!) a substitution for professional medical assistance. In this book we say repeatedly that if an injury or illness is serious, the victim should be carried out as soon as possible and in a safe way.

What's the difference then between wilderness first aid and regular first aid? If you're performing WFA, you're somewhere in the wilderness; you don't have the option usually of calling the hospital to send an ambulance. In fact, professional medical care may be a long way away—hours or even days. When you're administering WFA, you're also dealing with the elements. You may have to splint an arm in a blinding rainstorm or bandage a severe cut during heavy snow. It's also possible you'll have to perform these and other actions at high altitudes or in other inhospitable conditions. As you spend more time in the wilderness, you'll start to recognize that some kinds of physical injuries happen more often—for instance, it's not uncommon for people hiking to come in contact with a poison plant or suffer hypothermia. Because it may take time for rescue or transport to be arranged, you will almost certainly have to do more than you would if you were providing traditional first aid.

Where this book differs greatly from other books and training courses designed for WFA is in the treatment of common injuries and ailments. Most courses are designed using industry-standard equipment made for first aid such as bandages, burn creams, activated charcoal, and SAM (structural aluminum malleable) splints. However, the typical outdoorsman does not carry such items on a regular basis.

Therefore, this book has been designed to make use of items found within the typical outdoorsman's daypack as well as those found in nature. We call these items the Ten Cs—the items that anyone planning to go outdoors for hours or more at a time should have in case of an emergency or survival situation. With these ten simple items and the addition of medicinal plants, you will be able to effectively manage the most common injuries and ailments that occur in the outdoors. See "The Ten Cs" discussion in Chapter 2 for more information.

By preparing and practicing ahead of time, you'll be ready to cope in the event of a medical emergency.

Chapter 1

KNOW BEFORE
YOU GO

"Nature never deceives us; it is always we who deceive ourselves."

—Jean-Jacques Rousseau

You're walking along a trail when you nearly step on a snake. It darts out its head and bites you on the leg. What should you do?

You're at camp chopping firewood for your evening campfire. The axe slips and gashes your leg. How can you stop the bleeding?

While cooking dinner over the fire, you pick up a hot pan and burn your hand. What's the best treatment?

These are all situations you may encounter in the wilderness, and all of them require knowledge of first-aid techniques. But treating injuries and illnesses in the wild isn't something you should attempt without a little planning and education. Being prepared means you are more likely to stay calm and to do the right thing.

DEVELOP AN EMERGENCY PLAN

You've probably had a discussion with your family about what to do in the case of a fire, tornado, or hurricane—emergencies that may happen at home. You should create a similar emergency plan for when you're in camp:

- Let people back home know where you'll be and when you're expected back—so that if you don't show up, they'll know something's wrong.
- Create a buddy system to help prevent someone from wandering off from the group, especially if you'll have children with you.
- Get to know the general area where you'll be staying and agree on where you'll meet if members of your group will be splitting up.
- Check the forecast and agree on what to do if extreme weather comes along.
- Find out how to get to the nearest first-aid station, ranger station, or hospital before you do anything else and have an understanding of how long it may take for those responders to reach you in the area you've chosen to explore.
- Ensure each person, including youths, are carrying emergency gear and are familiar with how to use it.

HANDLING STRESS

Anyone who's been injured while out in the wild knows that all the stress you feel in such a situation is magnified. You're a long way from civilization, there's no doctor around, and you're struggling with pain (and quite possibly a significant trauma either in the form of blood loss or something else). It's well known that psychological and emotional stress can complicate and aggravate the physical symptoms of an injury. Those involved may also feel guilt for having contributed in some way to the emergency or for not preventing it. This is particularly so if the injured person is a friend or family member.

When the injured party is a close friend or family member, we often act in one of two ways: we don't take the injury or illness as seriously as perhaps we should because we know the person so well and expect him to "suck it up," or we overreact and create unnecessary panic at the presence of what we believe to be an abnormal amount of blood lost or deformation of a limb. If you're the one administering first aid, be reassuring and calm. You can communicate this to the victim by your manner as well as your words.

Applying this mentality to everyone, even those closely related to you, will prevent you from panicking. Losing your calm is the worst thing you could do as it may lead to you making poor decisions or feeling as if you can't act at all. If you train ahead of time, you will feel more confident when an emergency arises.

In an emergency situation, take a few deep breaths and concentrate on what you need to do right now to solve the problem. Making an immediate plan of action will help you focus and get your mind off fearful thoughts. Don't worry about what will happen tomorrow or next week.

In a group, it is common for one person's panic to spread to others. If the person panicking is not the injured party, ask him to take some deep breaths and calm down. Appoint another person to help keep the group calm. If this doesn't work or you don't have time, you may need to ask the panicking person to leave the area. In general, if you stay calm, it will help others around you stay calm.

If the person panicking is the injured party, you will need to calm him down as you give treatment. Encourage deep breaths (if appropriate) and help him focus on the positives of the situation instead of dwelling on worst-case scenarios. If possible, ask another group member to help keep the injured person calm. Tell the person involved what you're doing. Don't be dismissive, since the victim is in pain and may be in shock. You want to project an air of calm, reassurance, and competence.

If the injured person is conscious and understands what's going on, ask her for opinions about her treatment. You don't always have to follow her recommendations, but the more she's involved in the decisions you make about her care, the more she'll be comfortable with what you're doing.

INFECTIOUS DISEASE PRECAUTIONS

Keep in mind that when you're giving first aid to someone, you're in some danger of being infected. Viruses and bacteria live in blood and saliva and can give you such diseases as hepatitis, tuberculosis, pneumonia, and hard-to-treat skin infections.

For this reason, check your hands to make sure you don't have any open wounds or sores before beginning the physical examination of the victim. If the victim is coughing, keep your face away from him and try to avoid breathing in any sputum. Germs are tiny, but they can be deadly, and it's best to assume that the person you're treating is capable of infecting you unless you take precautions.

But how are you going to treat an injury if you can't touch the victim? The same way a doctor does: by insulating yourself from the patient. Of course, you don't have a surgical gown and mask, but the most important thing you can use is nitrile gloves. In your first-aid kit also pack some protective glasses or goggles and a couple of face masks. If you don't have these items, use trash bags or sandwich bags in place of gloves and improvise safety glasses using sunglasses or reading glasses. You can tie a bandanna around the lower part of your face and mouth to serve as a mask against germs.

HELPING AS A TEAM

When you are with a group and an accident or illness occurs, it's important for one person to take charge to prevent confusion. If there is a designated group leader or medic, you should follow that person's directions. When there isn't a group leader—such as on an outing with friends—the task of dealing with the emergency usually falls to the person who is keeping a level head. If that's you, then don't be afraid to take charge and to assign roles to other group members.

If the emergency is serious, one person should be tasked with organizing evacuation while someone else treats the injury. If possible, another person should be assigned the role of helping the caregiver. This might mean fetching supplies or keeping the injured person calm.

PRACTICAL SCENARIO

Let's say you go on a mission trip with your local church. You know those on the trip fairly well, but they're not your closest friends. One day during your outing through the jungle of Honduras, one of your teammates suffers a cut on his arm from a machete. The cut is bleeding pretty seriously. You know that direct pressure can help slow or stop the bleeding, but your first-aid kit and the team medic are miles away in another village. What do you do?

ANSWER

Irrigate the wound with potable water to clear away any debris such as plant material. When a proper irrigation syringe is not available, remember: the solution to pollution is dilution. This means you flood the area with clean water to flush out debris. You then remove any imbedded material such as dirt or bark by using the tip of your knife blade, a multitool, or even a toothpick.

Once the area is cleaned, apply a clean cotton dressing over the wound such as a bandanna or T-shirt, followed by firm direct pressure for the next fifteen minutes. Elevating the arm will also help stop bleeding. After fifteen minutes, check the wound to see if bleeding has slowed or stopped. If it has slowed, you may continue to apply direct pressure for another fifteen minutes or create a pressure dressing by tying another piece of material over the wound, making sure the knot or tightest part of the tied material is placed over the injured area. This will free up your hands so you can further treat the injury if necessary or help with evacuation.

If the bleeding has stopped, reinforce the dressing by adding more. Immobilize the limb so that it does not flail about and is not in danger of being bumped during evacuation, which could cause the wound to open again. (See Chapter 6 for details on creating an immobilization device in the wilderness.)

Knowing the person doesn't change the need for infectious disease precautions.

FIRST AID FOR YOURSELF

Imagine . . .

You're out by the lake alone at dawn when you accidentally stick the fishhook through your hand. Or you're hiking with friends but they get ahead while you're exploring a side trail. You slip and fall, twisting your ankle. You're hurt and you're on your own. Now what?

These are fairly frequent occurrences among outdoorsmen. So it's crucial to know how to take care of yourself.

First aid when applied to yourself is known as self-aid and should be considered the cornerstone of your first-aid training. After all, if you cannot properly care for yourself, why would you think you could care for someone else? Worse yet, if you and a friend both get injured, knowing how to care for yourself so that you can also care for your friend is a vital skill.

When *you're* the injured person, it's crucial for you to remain calm and act rationally because a momentary lapse in judgment could create a dangerous situation that you may not be able to address in a remote location without proper medical care.

While the treatments for various injuries and illnesses are the same whether you're treating yourself or someone else, treating yourself adds a level of complexity to the process. You're in pain, your mobility may be limited (you can only use one hand to get the fishhook out of your other hand), and you can only do one thing at a time. Throughout this book, sidebars will give additional information for treating injuries when they've happened to you.

The most important thing to remember is to keep calm. Then, assess the situation and make a plan. Can you call for help first, or do you need to stop the bleeding before doing anything else? Are you safe where you are or do you need to get to a more secure location before treating yourself? Though it can be challenging, with knowledge and the right attitude, you can give yourself appropriate first-aid treatment for many common emergencies.

SELF-AID

Remember one important thing: most of us begin any journey dehydrated to some degree. That's because the majority of us do not drink enough water daily. The chance of becoming ill from dehydration only increases when you are performing other tasks or caring for someone else and you forget the simplest preventative measures.

You should drink 64 ounces of water per day under normal circumstances. This volume increases with physical activity. If your urine isn't clear or pale yellow, you're already dehydrated to some degree (unless you're on a medication or vitamin that colors your urine). If you're not urinating at least every two hours, it's a sign that you are already dehydrated. This simple issue gets more students at our bushcraft school into trouble than any other single factor.

REDUCING THE LIKELIHOOD OF ILLNESS

While much of the material in this book focuses on accidents and injuries, being ill in the great outdoors can be dangerous, too. While you'll survive a case of the sniffles even without a nasal decongestant and chicken soup, a bout with pneumonia may cause a lot more trouble.

Just because you're in the wilderness doesn't mean you should be any less clean-conscious than if you were in your home. Wash your hands before eating, keep your utensils and dishes clean, and be sure to wash your hands after going to the toilet.

Check food before you eat it to make it hasn't gone off. Getting a case of food poisoning in the wild will really put a crimp in your trip. If you need certain medications, make sure you have them with you, as well as a backup supply that you can easily get to if your daypack gets lost overboard when your canoe capsizes.

TIPS AND TRICKS

- Wood ash makes an excellent soap substitute. Use it to wash your hands to kill bacteria and eliminate odors. You may also use it to powder your feet or use it under your arms for the same purpose and use it to powder your thighs if you are prone to chafing.
- Give yourself a limited window of time to be late back home— no more than three hours. In the event you do become seriously injured, the sooner someone comes looking, the better.
- Pour out 1 cup, 1 liter, and 2 liters of colored water on a hard surface such as your driveway, then on the ground so you become familiar with blood loss amounts and what they look like. Depending on how big you are, your body has between 4.5 and 5.5 liters of blood. Lose a quarter of it, and you could die.

- If you are exerting yourself a lot and not resting properly, your immune system will suffer. Carry Emergen-C packets or a similar vitamin C supplement, or make pine needle tea from shortleaf pines to add vitamin C to your system as an immune booster.

Chapter 2

SURVIVAL SKILLS FOR THE WILDERNESS

"The more injuries you get, the smarter you get."
—Mikhail Baryshnikov

Many times injury and illness in the wilderness can be prevented with proper preparation. If you have planned appropriately, packed your kit effectively, and understand the risks, you can often avoid emergency situations. The best treatment is prevention! With that in mind, let's look at some of the most important things you can do to prevent injury and illness.

THE TEN CS

The Ten Cs are the basic tools that an outdoors person should always take with her or him. The first five items are considered the most important because they are the most difficult to re-create in the wilderness. With the proper learning curve and skill level, you should be able to re-create the last four Cs of the first five with your first tool, the knife.

The Pathfinder System was developed by Dave Canterbury, one of this book's authors, who has more than twenty years of bushcrafting, outdoor self-reliance, and primitive-skills experience. As a hunting guide and experimental archaeology buff, Dave started thinking about what a person should have with him and what he should do in case of emergency. He sifted through archaeological and academic journal resource materials to discover what items were common cross-culturally among people who lived from the landscape. He put in the time, testing the skills and equipment, and developed the Pathfinder System. This system trains the beginner or experienced outdoorsman, bushcrafter, or adventurer in outdoor self-reliance, primitive skills, and survival skills. The system is designed for anyone who wants to learn these skills: the hunter, fisherman, trapper, hiker, search and rescue (SAR) and law enforcement professionals, or anyone who enjoys the outdoors. You never know when you may become lost or stranded, and with the invaluable skills taught by the Pathfinder System, you can survive an emergency situation. The Ten Cs are part of this system. More about the Pathfinder System can be found in *Bushcraft 101*.

The first five (most important) items are:

1. Cutting tool (knife)
2. Combustion device (ferrocerium rod, cigarette lighter, or magnification lens)
3. Container (stainless steel bottle or canteen)
4. Cordage (bank line or paracord)
5. Cover (emergency survival blanket or 3-millimeter-thick, 55-gallon drum liner)

With these five items alone you can effectively overcome, with some effort, adverse outdoor conditions. When applied to first-aid use, these items give you a way to create a shelter, treat shock, make splints and tourniquets, control bleeding, boil water, irrigate wounds, and more.

The remaining five items are designated as comfort items. While not comfortable in the traditional sense, these items make survival a little easier.

1. Cotton material (3' × 3' cloth or bandanna)
2. Candling device (headlamp)
3. Compass (orienteering style with mirror and magnification lens)
4. Cargo tape (Gorilla Tape)
5. Combination tool (multitool including an awl)

With these remaining items, you gain the ability to work in low-light conditions, find your way, make bandages and dressings, close wounds, treat minor burns, and much more.

By mixing these core kit items with a little ingenuity and bushcraft skill, you will learn to treat common injuries in the wilderness and better aid in the process of rescue and evacuation.

DRESSING FOR SURVIVAL

Among the most important things in preparing to go into the wilderness is to make sure that you're wearing appropriate clothing. Here are some basic tips:

- The best fiber to wear is wool, especially if you're camping in one of the colder months. It can absorb water without feeling wet immediately and it'll continue to protect you from the cold. Wool that's tight woven will keep you warmer than synthetic fibers.
- Generally avoid cotton. As soon as it gets wet it loses any insulative qualities, and in any case it's not going to keep you

very warm. However, if you're going to be hiking in a desert or some other dry, hot place, cotton is a good option. You can drench your T-shirt, and it will keep you cool while the water evaporates.

- One great advantage of synthetic fibers is that they don't absorb as much water as cotton or nylon; they also dry much faster than natural fibers. That said, they can be hazardous to wear near a fire, since the fabric might melt and burn you.

LAYERING

When outdoors, dressing in layers helps you stay protected even as the weather changes. The heavy long-sleeved shirt that was the right choice in the dawn hours could become quite uncomfortable under a blazing noontime sun; the T-shirt that was fine for eating lunch at a picnic table can turn out to be a bad idea when a sudden rain shower moves in.

Layering also gives you flexibility as you perform various activities throughout the day. The sweatshirt that was the right choice for quietly fishing under the shade of an oak tree might be too heavy for a vigorous hike, making it more likely that you'll overheat and potentially cause a medical problem.

By layering, you can easily put on or take off clothing as needed to suit your current circumstances. Think in threes: an inner layer, a middle layer, and an outer layer. The inner layer is generally a lightweight fabric that keeps moisture (sweat) away from your skin to help you stay comfortable. The middle layer provides insulation and some protection from the elements (for example, a long-sleeved shirt that keeps the sun and bugs off your skin). The outer layer protects you from water and wind.

In the summer months, the inner layer might be a T-shirt, the middle layer might be a lightweight long-sleeved shirt, and the outer layer might be a lightweight rain jacket. In winter, the middle layer could consist of several pieces of clothing to help you stay warm. In terms of insulation, it is generally better to have more layers instead of thicker layers; the air trapped between each layer contributes to the insulating value of your clothing. See Figure 2.1.

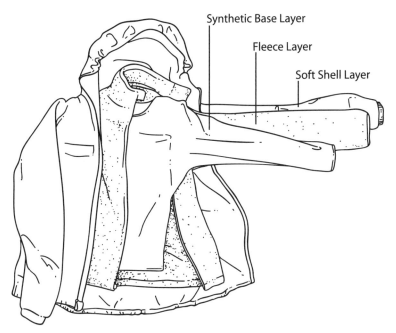

Synthetic Base Layer

Fleece Layer

Soft Shell Layer

Figure 2.1. Example of a three-layer alpine clothing system

FIVE-MINUTE FIRE

Fire can mean the difference between life and death in an emergency situation. Weather conditions will affect fire making, and being able to produce a sustainable fire with marginal materials in a variety of weather conditions is an important skill.

THE SURE-FIRE FIRE STARTER

We recommend that you carry a "sure-fire" fire-starting product such as Mini Inferno or Micro Inferno. Natural sure-fire tinders include pine-resin-laden fatwoods and birch barks. Even if they're wet, these kinds of tinders will burn and help you get a fire going, even if some of the firewood and kindling is damp.

We also recommend that you carry several methods of sparking a fire. The traditional cigarette lighter will fail in extremely cold or wet and windy conditions, but a ferrocerium rod, which is made of various mischmetals (an alloy of rare earth metals) and magnesium, will provide thousands of strikes in any weather condition with a shower of sparks as hot as 3,000°F. See Figure 2.2.

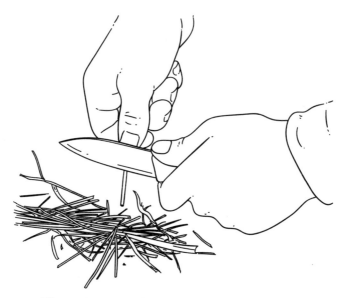

Figure 2.2. A student striking a ferro rod with the back of a knife blade

Your objective for WFA and survival purposes is to be able to create a sustainable fire in five minutes or less. A sustainable fire is a fire that is burning fuel of at least 1" in diameter, which means you can walk away for a moment and not fear the fire suddenly going out. There are many reasons you want to be able to make a fire within five minutes, but the most common is for hypothermia prevention. The longer it takes to make the fire in hypothermic conditions, the harder it will be to make, as your body will begin to shut down. That also means potentially crucial time will be lost before you can rewarm frostbitten extremities and drink water, which may need to be boiled first.

TINDER SELECTION

Tinder selection is important when it comes to making a fire quickly. Tinder is not your "sure-fire"; it is a means to effect sure-fire. Ideally tinder is dry natural material from the surrounding landscape. Cedar bark, fibrous plants, tall dead grasses, pine needles, and wood shavings are all viable options. Kindling is comprised of sticks ranging in size from the diameter of pencil lead up to about 1" thick. This is the material you will use to create fast, intense heat to combust your fuel sticks. The amount of kindling you collect should be about the size of a basketball, a pile you could carry under your arm.

BUILDING A BIRD'S NEST

The first step is to create a "bird's nest" with these materials. Your sure-fire device is the "egg" in the center. The size of the nest will vary depending on your experience level, but for true emergency situations such as survival or WFA, remember, "As big as your head, or your fire is dead." This means you want a bird's nest as big as your face to give your sure-fire the best conditions possible to create a decent flame capable of combusting your kindling. See Figure 2.3.

Avoid putting on more fuel until the flames reach a height of at least 2" above what's currently burning. This will happen quickly if you have laid your fire properly. Once this occurs, you're ready to add your fuel sticks, and you are on your way to having a sustainable fire capable of staving off hypothermia, boiling water, and much more.

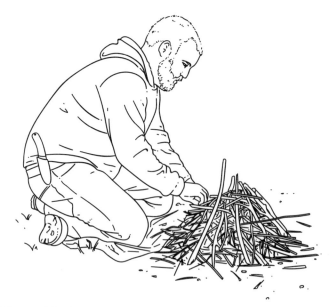

Figure 2.3. A student with kindling placed over bird's nest

Practice makes perfect, and fire making is something you've got to be good at in the wild. The more you work at it, under different conditions and at different times of the year, the better you'll get. At the heart of fire making is understanding what the fire needs—is it fuel or oxygen? Spend time before you build your fire thinking about the optimum place to put it. It should be far enough from your shelter not to pose a fire hazard but not so far away that you can't easily utilize it and tend to it.

FIVE-MINUTE SHELTER

Besides fire, a well-constructed shelter is essential for survival in the wild. It can take just a few hours of exposure for the body to begin exhibiting symptoms of hypothermia (too cold) or hyperthermia (too hot)—and it doesn't take more than a few minutes to risk sunburn or frostbite. It's essential to know how to quickly create some sort of shelter. Not only will you be shielded from snow or rain, you can also control—to some extent—the temperature inside, which is important when treating injuries such as frostbite.

An important item in your pack in this regard is an All-Weather Emergency Blanket or SOL Emergency Blanket. Using a rope, create a ridgeline between two trees. The rope should be at waist height. Then attach the front corners of the blanket to the rope and secure the rear corners on the ground. Now you have a lean-to in which you can move the patient. Make sure to place the reflective side of the blanket down to maximize heat retention. See Figure 2.4.

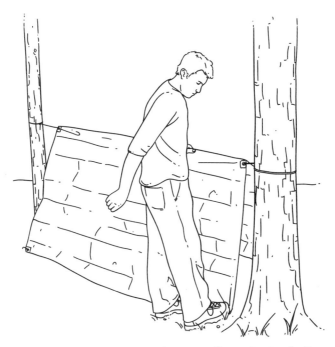

Figure 2.4. A student setting up a five-minute shelter

Since in most circumstances it will be important to keep the patient warm, build a fire one large step directly in front of the shelter (make sure the flames don't come in contact with the blanket).

Construct a reflecting wall from rocks or logs behind the fire. If your object is to get the patient into a cooler environment, turn the reflective side of the blanket outward.

FIVE-MINUTE WATER BOIL

After you have set up a shelter and started a fire, the next step is to boil water as quickly as possible so you have potable water to treat injuries and rewarm and feed the victim. You don't have much time here. Fortunately it's pretty simple to boil water quickly if you know what you're doing. Fill a container with water (stainless steel bottle or canteen). Take off the lid and use the stove base or a couple of green sticks (wood that has been recently cut and hasn't dried out, making it less likely to burn) to raise the container about 2" off the ground.

Doing this will permit air to pass under the container and help it to superheat. Prop sticks over the container, imitating a tepee, and surround the container with more kindling. This will also help heat the water quickly.

Once the water has boiled, allow it to cool. Hanging it from a toggle will help speed this process.

In all, all of the steps listed here (building a shelter, building a fire, boiling water) shouldn't take you more than fifteen minutes; with some practice you can probably get it down to seven or eight. Spend the time mastering these skills. They can save a life in the wilderness.

COMMON OUTDOOR INJURIES AND ACCIDENTS

Many common outdoor injuries and accidents could be prevented with planning. Some of the most common problems are:

- **Breaks, sprains, and strains.** Falls are a common cause of injury, especially when crossing uneven or rocky areas. You don't even have to fall to break an ankle—sometimes just a misstep will do the trick. The National Institutes of Health reports that about 70 percent of all nonfatal wilderness injuries are breaks, sprains, and strains. Make sure you have appropriate footwear, and don't be in a rush when conditions are wet or otherwise dangerous. Don't hike in the dark, and do ankle- and knee-strengthening exercises before you set out.

- **Weather-related illnesses.** Hypothermia and hyperthermia can be prevented with proper clothing and shelter, plenty of fresh, clean water to drink, and a careful eye on the weather forecast.
- **Sunburns and rashes.** Use a good sunscreen and apply it frequently throughout the day—you can get sunburned even in winter months if you're outside all day. Don't touch plants with bare skin unless you're sure they're not poison ivy or another plant that will leave you itching.

BUSHCRAFT TIP

According to the National Institutes of Health, falls and drowning are the most common causes of death for people exploring the wilderness. Use special care when hiking and climbing and when near water.

USING PROPER GEAR AND TECHNIQUES

Accidents and injuries commonly occur when people use incorrect gear and techniques to perform a task. For example, when striking a ferro rod, do so with the back of your knife, not the blade. Using the blade risks a bad cut should the knife or the rod slip.

Reduce the likelihood of injuries by always keeping cutting tools sharp; dull tools have a tendency to slip and do more damage. Keep sharp tools properly covered, using masks for axes and sheathes for knives. Never leave them lying about your camp location unprotected. Take care to choose your footing wisely while on the trail, and clear trip hazards from your working area while in camp.

Wear proper protective clothing. In spring and summer it can be tempting to wear shorts and a T-shirt but (depending on what you'll be doing) it could be asking for injury and infection. Always overdress with protective long pants and sleeves so that you can adjust to the environment. This will also help prevent sunburn. A wide-brimmed hat will be an asset to you on many occasions, such as during sudden rain or on extremely sunny days.

To understand how to use your gear correctly and sharpen your skills, practice at home before you go off into the wilderness. Mistakes will be less dangerous and easier to correct.

STAYING SAFE WHILE IMPROVISING

That said, half of the fun of being outdoors is learning how to improvise—to make use of what's at hand instead of trekking it all in. The key is in knowing how to improvise safely, which means understanding your materials and the environment.

For example, you may think that setting your kettle on a rock in the middle of your fire means you won't have to carry in a campfire tripod, but a wet rock placed in a fire can explode. Spend some time learning about the environment before you put it to work.

KNOW YOUR LIMITS

Being an outdoorsman often means pushing yourself to do more than you thought you could do. But going past your limits is a common cause of injury and illness. "Just one more mile" in the bitter cold can lead to hypothermia, and "I think I can jump across this creek" can lead to a bad fall. Knowing what your physical limits are can help you enjoy your wilderness experience instead of suffering through it.

Preparing ahead of time (for example, by doing strength- and endurance-building exercises) can help. If you must push your limits, make sure a buddy is with you in case you need help.

TIPS AND TRICKS

- Quaking aspen trees produce a chalky dust called bloom that is useful for sunscreen with an SPF of about 5. It has been documented as being traditionally used by Native Americans.
- Bic-style cigarette lighters will generally fail in temperatures less than 32°F. This makes a good temperature gauge. The lighter can be made usable easily enough by warming it with body heat for a few minutes.
- You will see your breath at 40°F. This can help you gauge how cold it is.
- Punk woods from soft trees in the aspen family will readily ignite to an ember with a magnification lens as long as the materials are dry.
- You can easily insulate the ground inside an emergency shelter by stuffing a 55-gallon drum liner with dry materials such as weeds and grasses and compressing it into a flat layer about 4" thick.
- Wearing boots that do not lace can be a blessing in disguise to many folks: there is less chance of getting poison ivy on the hands, they are easier to put on and remove if one hand or arm is injured, and if you get your boot stuck in mud or rocks for some unfortunate reason, you can slip the foot out.

— Chapter 3 —

THE EMERGENCY SCENE

"Injuries obviously change the way you approach the game."

—BRETT FAVRE

When you need to give first aid to someone in a wilderness setting, often you know exactly what happened and how because you were there when it occurred. But sometimes you don't know—your friend is off gathering firewood when you hear a shout, or perhaps you come across someone sitting by the side of the trail you're hiking up. In those cases, you don't always know what has happened or how, so you need to assess the situation before trying to treat the injured or ill person.

FIRST APPROACH

When you're walking toward someone who's been hurt, it's only natural if you feel your heart beat faster and your palms start to sweat. It's a very stressful situation, and your body is producing adrenaline to help you cope. What you've got to do is internally talk yourself down. There's no good reason to rush, and doing so may cause more harm than good. Stop if necessary to take a couple of deep breaths and remind yourself that you're there to help.

If you don't know the person, take a moment to introduce yourself and ask permission to help. Tell him or her that you're trained. The more you can do at this early stage to induce confidence in the victim, the easier your job will be.

As you approach, survey the scene to make sure there are no hazards that could affect you and to look for what caused the injury.

LOOK AROUND YOU

Unless you stay safe, you won't be able to help others in their time of need, and you may suffer a serious injury yourself. While counting slowly to ten, look all around you, taking in as much detail as possible. Something as simple as twisting your ankle can mean you lose the ability to help the injured person. Leaning trees, loose limbs overhead, loose or falling rock, water hazards, animal hazards, hazardous materials, and storm hazards are some of the most common issues.

The world isn't going to stand still while you're administering first aid. All kinds of things can happen: other people may come on the scene and want to help; animals may show up to investigate; or weather conditions may suddenly change. This can interfere with your continued safety (and that of the person you are treating). So throughout your time on the scene, continue re-evaluating it.

For example, if you find that a swarm of hornets is buzzing about an unconscious person, you may not be able to approach her right away without succumbing to multiple stings, which could lead to your own emergency situation. Similarly, if you determine that a patient has been struck by a widow maker (a broken-off treetop or limb) and you identify more in the area, you should move the injured person out of harm's way before beginning your assessment since one gust of wind the wrong way could lead to another widow maker falling—this time on you!

PRACTICAL SCENARIO

As you're hiking along your favorite trail, you notice an individual lying across the trail, apparently unconscious. As you continue your approach, you shout out, asking if he's okay while scanning the area for obvious hazards such as fallen limbs and loose debris signifying he may have tripped and fallen or obvious animal sign. You detect an unnatural odor of cucumber in the air. Upon reaching the patient, you notice two punctures on his ankle—denoting a snake bite. What should you do?

ANSWER

Certain snakes such as the copperhead emit a musk when touched. A strong odor of cucumber, which is what this musk resembles, would indicate the snake is still in the vicinity. So, your first reaction should be to inspect your surroundings and carefully move the injured person in case the snake has taken refuge under his collapsed body. In the event you cannot locate the snake but still perceive it to be close, it may be a good idea to move the person a short distance away to safety before administering first aid.

RESCUING AN INJURED PERSON

Sometimes an injured person is in a situation requiring rescue, not just treatment. For example, if a hiker has been hurt by a falling tree limb, he or she might still be trapped under it. Or, in a more dire scenario, you might recognize that someone is drowning and needs to be pulled out of the water.

- First, remember that you should never jeopardize your own safety to help someone else.
- Call for help if possible.
- Be aware that "rescue action" and "giving first aid" are two different things under the law. If by rescuing a person (for

example, pulling him out of a vehicle after an accident), you create or worsen an injury, that is different from potentially causing or worsening an injury while giving treatment (for example, if the tourniquet you apply is too tight). While Good Samaritan laws can protect you in the latter case, they won't necessarily protect you in the former.

- Don't move an injured person until you've had a chance to determine the extent of her injuries, unless the hazard of leaving her is potentially life-threatening.

- Sometimes treatment and rescue have to happen at the same time. For example, the pressure of a tree limb that has trapped an injured person's leg might be minimizing the bleeding. When it is moved, the bleeding will worsen, and you will need to take immediate action to stop it.

- If you suspect someone in the water is in distress and possibly drowning, remember that your first move shouldn't be to jump in the water yourself to save him. If you can reach him without being pulled into the water yourself (hold on to something stable), try that. Or, throw him a flotation device to hold on to. If neither of those options will work, row or swim out to the person using some sort of flotation device (an inner tube, a canoe).

BUSHCRAFT TIP

People who are near to drowning don't splash around in the water calling for help (although a tired or distressed swimmer may do this). Someone in the state of *active* drowning can't even reach for a nearby flotation device. Signs of active drowning include the head being low in the water and tilted back, eyes closed or glassy (not focusing), and not using the legs. The most counterintuitive aspect of drowning is that the swimmer may not seem in distress. If you suspect someone is in trouble, ask, "Are you all right?" If the swimmer can answer, she is probably okay. If not, then she needs help.

MECHANISM OF INJURY

While you're looking around the area where the person was injured, try to pinpoint the particular things that caused the injury. For instance, you may see some fallen rocks that struck the victim. Or you may notice a clump of poison sumac that the person came into contact with. Weather can be a factor as well. Assessing *how* the injury happened ("mechanism of injury") can help you determine what the injury actually is and how serious it is likely to be.

Even a short fall—for example, from 3'—can do serious harm. When someone falls more than three times his own height, he's probably injured his spine. If the victim has suffered blunt trauma above the clavicles, it's very possible she's injured her cervical spine. Therefore, someone who falls and hits her head could also have damaged her cervical spine.

Remember to keep animals and insects as part of your calculations. If the victim disturbed a hive of yellow jackets and suffered multiple stings, the area is probably still hazardous. The same is true of bites from an animal. In these cases, your first priority is to get the victim away from the site of the injury. You may first have to wait out the animal or insect swarm before you enter the scene. An enraged animal or swarm will seek to defend its den or area, which will likely result in you becoming injured yourself. If there is an opportunity to remove the injured person from the active site, do so as long as it does not put you in immediate danger.

Use your common sense when evaluating the mechanism of injury. Remember the old adage, "If you hear hoofbeats, think horses, not zebras." Someone sitting by the trail holding her ankle probably isn't suffering a heart attack.

By the same token, if the injuries don't seem congruent with what you would expect, then take a mental step back and reassess. For example, if someone has taken a fall and you expect skinned knees and maybe a sprained ankle, but he is vomiting blood, something else has happened.

Determining the mechanism of injury is the detective portion of the scene assessment. By evaluating clues both objective and subjective you can determine the course of immediate care.

PRACTICAL SCENARIO

You are driving your four-wheeler on a trail and you find a side-by-side collision at an intersection of the trail. Three people are out walking around the accident scene. As you approach the scene, you see there is considerable intrusion into the front end of one of the vehicles with a badly bent frame. You also notice there is a rear passenger compartment wherein a crying boy is being cared for by his father, neither of whom is wearing a helmet. You discover that the other three individuals are two hikers and the driver of the other vehicle, whom you are told is "fine." What should be your first course of action?

ANSWER

The first thing you should do is appoint someone to call 911. One of the hikers is ideal since they are not directly involved in the emergency. What type of injuries might you expect to find in an ATV collision in which the occupants were not wearing helmets and one vehicle suffered significant frame damage? Likely injuries to the head, neck, spine, hands, arms, and knees, and potential blunt force trauma to the thoracic cavity.

Because there is a child involved, with a parent already providing some sort of care, you naturally begin your assessment there and find that the child banged his head against the front seat and is bleeding from a gash in the forehead, has some blood on the lips, and is having trouble catching his breath. As you further assess the child, the smell of alcohol becomes apparent from the father, who seems to be emotionally shaken and has a knot on his forehead, labored breathing, and abnormally distended neck veins.

As you make this assessment, ask: are there any other hazards to consider? Is there smoke or a smell of gasoline? Is the engine still running or is the vehicle in an unsteady and precarious position? Is there a need for a modified triage system to screen for hidden injuries?

> The loudest victim is not always the one in need of immediate assistance. The fact that the boy is crying tells us his airway is open and that he is vocal. A well-trained aid giver would more thoroughly consider the mechanism of injury. In this case, the father and son's vehicle was without airbags and they were not wearing helmets. The front-seat victim, given the significant mechanism of injury (front-end impact with bent frame), should receive a higher initial priority until injuries are completely ruled out. Therefore it would be better to assess the father and then the crying child. The other driver, who is walking around, should be last on your assessment list. All of this assessment occurs within the first two minutes of your arrival to the scene.

WHERE TO BEGIN?

The first thing to do is to determine if the victim's injuries or illness is life-threatening. Examine the patient for trauma by checking vital signs (pulse, breathing, etc.) and seeing how responsive he is. After you've announced yourself, gently touch his shoulder (or some other noninjured body part) and ask if he's all right. Then, determine his level of responsiveness (LOR). The LOR checks the injured person's awareness and ability to communicate.

AVPU

In characterizing an injured or ill person's level of responsiveness, use the AVPU scale.

A = Alert: The person is alert and can speak with you intelligibly. She knows what happened, who she is, and where she is. A few minutes of amnesia after a serious injury are common, but the patient recovers her memory fairly quickly. An alert person will be able to inform you of her condition and describe her injury.

V = Verbal: The person responds to verbal stimuli. She responds to your voice and can answer you. On the other hand, if she grimaces or rolls away from you when you speak, you will need to investigate further and perform other tests.

P = Painful: The person responds to painful stimuli. If you pinch her skin, she reacts. Just as with verbal stimuli, a reaction to pain means that the injured person is responsive, albeit in a diminished capacity. The patient might require immediate treatment before she becomes unresponsive. Further testing may indicate potentially life-threatening conditions.

U = Unresponsive: The person doesn't respond to any stimuli. If unresponsive, the injured person cannot give you any information, so you must rely on your senses and the guidance of your assessment to treat any life-threatening injuries.

ABCS

Once a level of responsiveness is determined you can assess the injured person's ABCs, or airway, breathing, and circulation. The purpose of this assessment is to determine whether or not there are problems with the injured person's airway, to see if he is struggling to breathe, and to figure out if he is losing blood.

A = Airway: Look at the victim's throat for any blockages. In an unresponsive patient, open the mouth and look down into the throat to check for blockages such as blood, food, and spittle, which you may need to remove or manage. If he's talking to you, his airway is open, but it's possible he's having trouble breathing. Ask him if it hurts to take breaths. You may remove blockages by finger sweeping the mouth or turning the patient onto his side into a recovery position (see "Recovery Position" later in this chapter), which will at times allow the material to drain out of the mouth, thereby clearing the airway.

B = Breathing: Labored breaths and noise while breathing, such as rattling or gurgling, could indicate an internal injury. Wheezing/whistling may indicate a puncture to the thoracic cavity.

C = Circulation: If the victim is responsive, take her pulse at her wrist. If she's not responsive, take it at the neck. A normal pulse rate is between 60 and 100 beats per minute. Anything above or below these numbers signifies a medical emergency. Examine her for any significant bleeding, especially her arms and legs. If bleeding is occurring, apply pressure to control it and create a bandage or tourniquet.

VITAL SIGNS

When you're making your initial examination of the victim, one of the first things you'll do is check his vital signs. This means you'll establish his level of responsiveness, as we discussed previously. You'll also check his heart rate, breathing rate, how well his blood is flowing, his temperature, moisture, and skin color. This will give you an idea of his overall health and point you toward your next steps. Generally speaking, someone who is alert with a heart rate of 72, with cool, normal-colored skin, breathing fifteen times a minute is normal, whereas someone who responds to verbal stimuli with a heart rate of 42, with cool, clammy skin, breathing ten times a minute with wheezing is in need of immediate medical care. Changes in vitals over a period are indications of an alteration in the injured person's condition for the better or worse. When you're checking the patient, if possible jot down in a notebook or some other paper the vital signs you're measuring.

Heart Rate (Pulse)

If your patient is responsive, you can check her wrist for a pulse. If she's unresponsive or too young to understand what you're doing, check her neck. Just below the jaw there's a groove between her windpipe and her neck muscle. One or two fingertips on that spot will give you a pulse. Never reach across the injured person to take a carotid pulse, as the person (or a bystander) may become startled and defensive.

To take a pulse at the wrist, look for the groove at the base of the thumb. Gently press on the area using two fingertips.

A weak pulse is obviously harder to find, so you may need to put a bit more pressure on the artery with your fingers. Use the distal (downstream) finger to do so, but be careful not to press too hard.

A normal heart beats between 60 and 100 times per minute. Rather than listen an entire sixty seconds (at a point where every minute may count), count the number of beats in fifteen seconds and multiply by four. Is the heartbeat regular? Is it strong? If not, the situation may be life-threatening. Write the pulse rate in your field notes. Higher and lower pulse rates may signify certain medical conditions (which are discussed throughout this book), so having a written record will allow you to better track them.

Circulation

Next you want to determine how the victim's blood is flowing to his extremities—his hands and feet. Press down on the nail bed of one of his fingers. How long does it take for the nail to turn pink again? More than two seconds indicates a problem. (Note that this method works best on children less than six years old.)

Respiratory Rate

Just as your heart normally beats at a given rate, you breathe in and out a given number of times per minute. If your patient is breathing less than twelve times a minute, the situation is life-threatening and you may have to perform rescue breathing. If the patient isn't breathing often enough, other parts of the body aren't getting the oxygen they need, and permanent damage or death can result.

Put your hand on the victim's chest and watch it rise and fall for fifteen seconds. Multiply by four and you know the per-minute breath rate.

In an unresponsive patient, look, listen, and feel for breathing. Look for chest rise and fall, listen for air movement in the chest cavity, and feel for air movement from the nose or mouth and chest. As you did with the pulse, take note of the regularity and strength of the breathing. Adults should breathe between twelve and twenty times a minute.

Skin Tissue Color, Temperature, and Moisture
To check skin tissue color, look at the inner eyelids, lips, and nail beds. Normal skin should be warm and dry. Here are some other things to take note of:

- If the injured person's skin is cool and clammy, he may be suffering from shock or anxiety.
- Cold and moist skin means the body is losing heat.
- Cold and dry skin means the body is suffering from exposure to extreme cold.
- Hot and dry skin means high fever or heat exposure.
- Goose bumps accompanied by shivering, blue lips, and teeth chattering can mean dysfunction of the autonomic system, fear, exposure to cold, or pain.
- Pale skin may mean blood loss, shock, hypotension, or emotional distress.
- Cyanotic (bluish-gray) skin means lack of oxygen and inadequate breathing and heart function.
- Flushed (red) skin means exposure to heat or emotional excitement.
- Yellow (jaundiced) skin indicates inadequate liver function.
- Mottled (blotchy) skin is occasionally seen in patients with shock.

PRIORITIZING TREATMENT

If you encounter an emergency situation where more than one person is injured or ill, you have to decide which person to treat first. Triage, as this assessment process is called, helps you prioritize the most severe and time-urgent illnesses and injuries, treating and stabilizing them before you move on to helping those with less severe or time-urgent problems. Although your first instinct may be just to dive in and start helping, taking some time to make this assessment increases the likelihood of positive outcomes for everyone involved.

In order of importance are injuries that require *immediate* attention, those that require *urgent* attention, and those that require *moderate* attention. Death is the lowest priority, as there is nothing you can do to help.

- **Immediate attention.** First priority should be given to an injured or ill person who has airway blockage or breathing difficulties, severe or uncontrolled bleeding, or confusion or disorientation.
- **Urgent attention.** After treating anyone who requires immediate attention, treat those who require urgent attention. This would be any injured or ill person who has burns (but an open airway), major broken bones or multiple broken bones or similar injuries such as sprains or dislocations, and spinal injuries (including suspected spinal injuries).
- **Moderate attention.** After treating the more serious injuries or illnesses, you can turn your attention to helping those with less severe problems, including minor breaks or sprains, cuts, scrapes, and bruises.

PHYSICAL EXAM

Now you've come to the physical exam, one of the most important parts of administering first aid. The patient's expressions and sounds as you carry out the exam can be important diagnostic indications, so keep an eye on her face. You'll be looking not only for obvious existing injuries but also for any secondary ones—particularly in the cases where hard trauma has occurred.

This is no time to be polite or shy! Be thorough and don't hesitate about unbuttoning clothing. Look for injuries that may not be obvious but that are causing pain or discomfort.

> **BUSHCRAFT TIP**
>
> Remember that very often the pain of an injury or illness is accompanied by fear, which can be debilitating. Keep your manner calm and encouraging and don't use any sort of catastrophic language around the victim. At the same time, be honest—if a hiker's leg is broken, you're not doing him any favors by lying and saying it's fine. If you're worried that the victim may be panicked by the truth, move the conversation in another direction. By engaging the person in positive conversation you help alleviate stress and build confidence, which keeps both you and the patient calm.

START AT THE TOP

Start with the head. Run your hands over the skull. If there are places that are loose or gravel-like, it could be fractured and what you're feeling are bone fragments. Check if the patient is bleeding from the ears or nose, since this could be related to a skull fracture.

If clear fluid is coming from the skull, ears, or nose, there's almost certainly been a skull injury; the fluid is cerebrospinal fluid (CSF). To check this, dip the corner of a light-colored cloth in the fluid. If the patch dries surrounded by a yellow halo, you've confirmed it's CSF.

The victim's eyes may appear surrounded by dark patches, giving him a look as if he's put on too much eye makeup. This is because blood from the surrounding tissues is spreading to the tissues near the eyes. It may be accompanied by Battle's Sign, which will appear as bruising behind the ear, a sign of a basal skull fracture.

Check the pupils by briefly shining a flashlight in them. Do they react normally to the light? If one pupil is bigger than the other, this is a sign of brain injury.

Now check the mouth. Look to see if the tongue has been injured or bitten off. Are the teeth all still there? Teeth can break in a fall and cut the inside of the mouth. If that's the case, the flow of blood into the mouth can block the airway, creating breathing problems. Can the victim move his jaw? Is there swelling anywhere around the lower part of the head.?

Smell his breath. If you smell a fruity odor, it is a sign of ketoacidosis, an excess of acid in the blood due to an irregularity of insulin typically associated with diabetes.

BUSHCRAFT TIP

People with chronic diseases such as diabetes often wear or carry medical alert information. Look for tattoos and bracelets on the wrist, ankle, or neck. Check the wallet for a medical alert card.

UPPER BODY

Moving down from the head, the next area of examination is the shoulders and chest.

The collarbone is often broken during severe falls. See if the patient can move his arms without pain. If something beneath the skin of the shoulders looks lumpy or out of shape, there's a good chance the collarbone has been broken.

Ribs are another set of bones often subject to breakage. Ask the victim if it hurts to breathe. Stand behind him, placing a hand on either side of the rib cage and ask him to breathe deeply. Are the ribs normal to the touch? Is one side painful or does it not rise with breathing? If ribs are broken, it's possible that one of them (or something else) has pierced the chest wall. This is called a sucking chest wound and can be particularly dangerous, since untreated it will build up pressure until the lungs collapse.

If the patient is coughing up blood, this could signal any number of things, from bronchitis to some sort of chronic condition. If you're hiking at a high altitude, it could be a sign of high-altitude pulmonary edema, and you should get the patient to a lower altitude as soon as possible.

The heart is a muscle, and like all muscles it can be bruised. A severe bruise will cause bleeding in the pericardial sac, surrounding the heart. Although this condition is treatable, it's not one you, a nonprofessional, should attempt to deal with in the wild.

> **BUSHCRAFT TIP**
>
> Injuries to young children should always be taken very seriously, since it may take a day or so for them to show symptoms, particularly where heartbeat and breathing are concerned. Keep a careful eye out for this.

ABDOMEN AND PELVIS

The abdomen is next on the examination list. Envision the abdomen in four quadrants. You palpate (press) on each quadrant, feeling for distension (gas released due to organ damage) and rigidity (internal bleeding).

The liver can be vulnerable to injury, which can cause extensive internal bleeding. (This shouldn't come as a surprise, since the function of the liver is to process your blood.)

If your patient is vomiting up blood, especially if it's mixed with bile, the liver has almost certainly been damaged. On the other hand, if the blood is mixed with spittle and digestive juices, the victim has been injured in her stomach. If it's bright red, it's coming from the esophagus.

After the accident, if the victim goes to the bathroom check (or have her check) her urine. If it contains blood, there's a chance her kidneys may have been injured. Any sort of internal bleeding issues are cause for concern, since the body will react by sharply contracting muscles, creating considerable pain. As well, the body's organs, when injured, will try to fight back by releasing microorganisms that can do damage to other parts of the body.

If the victim is pregnant and bleeding from the abdomen or vagina, the fetus or uterus may be injured.

Check the genital area as well; if the patient is male and has an uncontrolled erection after an accident, he may have suffered a spinal or pelvic injury.

The pelvis should be examined by pressing gently inward and downward on the pelvis bones to detect an injury.

ARMS AND LEGS

After the pelvis, check the legs. Press firmly around the upper bone of each leg (femur) and check for pain reaction. If it seems obvious to you that a part of the leg is injured (for instance, if you can see that the leg is bent at an unnatural angle), examine the rest of the leg first. When you're done, go back to the obvious injury. Pain in the surface tissue surrounding the femur may be so intense that the patient's muscles spasm (called guarding) or the patient refuses to allow you to properly palpate the leg to determine the extent of damage.

Feet are often the site of injuries because we put them through so much in the wild. When you're examining the victim's feet, look at circulation, indicated by their color, temperature, and pulse. The pulse is located in the hollow below and behind the inside ankle bone. If you have trouble finding that one, look between the two tendons on top of the foot. As with all pulses, you should feel them clearly and they should be strong and within normal limits of 60–100 beats per minute. A weak pulse can indicate a lag in blood flow to the extremity caused by interior blockage or exterior damage due to an injury.

See if the injured person can wiggle toes or apply upward and downward pressure with the feet. If the tissues of your feet freeze, you'll lose nerve function as well as circulation.

Follow this same process for the arms and fingers. Make a strength check by asking the victim to squeeze a couple of your fingers with each hand. If there is a difference between the two, one side may be injured or one side of the brain may be impaired, so further investigation may be required.

If there's no sign of a spinal injury, the next step is to log roll the patient to check her back for injuries. See "Moving an Injured Person" in this chapter for how to perform a log roll. Look for any injuries previously hidden such as blood loss from the back or any abnormalities such as deformities or impaled objects.

DCAP-BTLS

Many people find the DCAP-BTLS system helpful to remember what injuries you're searching for.

D = Deformities: Anything that should not appear on a healthy body
C = Contusions: Bruises
A = Abrasions: Scrapes, etc.
P = Punctures: Holes anywhere on the body
B = Burns: Redness, sunburn
T = Tenderness: Pain or muscle spasms in reaction to touch
L = Lacerations: Cuts
S = Swelling: Anywhere on the body

SELF-AID

You can also perform the examination techniques in this chapter on your own body if you have injured yourself and need to assess the damage. Write down your own vitals and keep track of them as you wait for help. Carry an XXL orange T-shirt within your kit as your cotton material. This item will fulfill all the functions of the cotton material and can also be worn over all your outerwear so you can be seen by a rescue team in the woods should you be immobile, sleeping, or unconscious.

SAMPLE HISTORY

If you're treating someone for a traumatic injury, the SAMPLE history isn't as useful and you can skip it. It's quite possible that the victim won't know all the answers to your questions, but you can get help from her friends and companions. As always, be calm and never be antagonistic. Your goal is to get information while keeping everyone calm. Make the questions open-ended and try to avoid questions to which the answer is yes or no.

S = Signs/symptoms: What signs of injury or illness have you found?

A = Allergies: Is the patient allergic to anything with which she could have come into contact?

M = Medications: Is the patient currently taking any medications, and if so, what for? Has she missed taking her dosage?

P = Pertinent medical history: Is there anything you and other first-aid providers should know about the patient?

L = Last oral intake: What was the last time the patient ate or drank anything? What was it?

E = Events: What led up to this situation? Was there a specific incident or have the symptoms come on slowly?

KEEP CHECKING

If your patient doesn't have any life-threatening injuries, you should check the ABCs and vital signs every fifteen minutes. This will enable you to make sure the patient is stable. Industry-standard protocol is to keep checking until care is transferred to EMS or other official medical provider. It's important to track any changes in the injured person's status. This is especially true if you suspect the patient has internal injuries such as bleeding, since the body will continue to react to those injuries and you may have to take further steps to stabilize the patient. However, should a person simply have a bruised elbow, it's easy enough to ask how he is feeling a few times per hour or until the initial onset of pain and swelling subsides. Let common sense prevail.

For patients with more substantial injuries such as fractured limbs, burns, or breathing problems due to wounds to the thoracic cavity, reassess every five minutes until additional help arrives.

MOVING AN INJURED PERSON

If someone's been severely hurt, your first concern should be to get him ready for evacuation. This is particularly true if he's sustained a neck or back injury, which makes moving him tricky. Your goal is to get him onto a backboard, which can support his body while you're moving him. To do this, the first step is to get him into what's called a neutral anatomical position. It's highly unlikely that you will re-create the damaging forces it took to injure the victim in the first place simply by moving him into a better position for transport, except in cases of falling from a significant height or being hit by something substantial, but take care to move deliberately and at a slow enough pace that current injuries are not worsened by jerky motions or unnatural rotations. In cases of falls from heights greater than 15' or impacts by large objects such as ATVs and trees, do not move the patient unless absolutely necessary until EMS arrives.

NEUTRAL ANATOMICAL POSITION

As you can see in Figure 3.1, a neutral anatomical position means the victim is lying on his back. His arms are at his side, and his feet are forward. One important concern at this point is to make sure that his airway doesn't have any blockages. You have already checked for this in your initial examination, but take a moment to confirm it. See Figure 3.1.

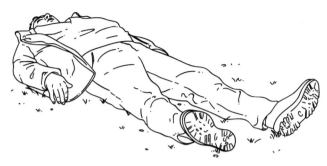

Figure 3.1. Neutral anatomical position

RECOVERY POSITION

A recovery position can be used when the victim isn't seriously injured. She should be placed on her side, with her head resting on her arm. She can bend her legs a bit to keep balanced. If she shows a tendency to vomit or cough blood and sputum, this is a good position, since the vomit and other excreta won't be able to block her airway. See Figure 3.2.

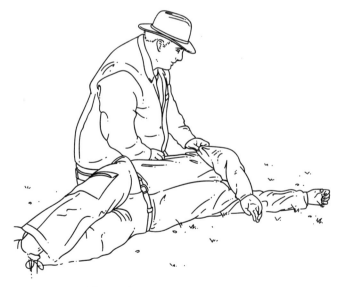

Figure 3.2. Recovery position

LOG ROLL

If you determine the injured person absolutely needs to be rolled on her side in order to be moved or to prevent choking, seek assistance if possible. The more people assisting, the better, because more hands can stabilize the injured person and prevent unwanted spinal motion. If you don't have help, you had better have a good reason to proceed with the log roll instead of waiting for EMS to arrive—such as an immediate life threat.

Generally at least two are needed for a safe log roll, one to stabilize the head and neck and one to stabilize the lower spine and pelvis. The person stabilizing the head and neck is the person in control, and he is the one who dictates when the roll occurs so that there is no confusion between parties resulting in an alternate twisting of the body.

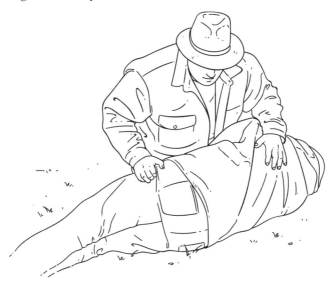

Figure 3.3. Log roll to check the back for injuries

The person at the head (#1) cradles the head and neck by placing hands at the ears and fingers under the neck while the second person (#2) positions her knees perpendicular to the patient allowing for the patient to be rolled toward her lap. Person #2 places her hands at the shoulder and hip of the patient and at the command of Person #1, pulls the patient in coordinated effort toward her lap, at which time a back assessment for bleeding and deformities is done. Then a backboard, blanket, or tarp is placed under the injured person before she is returned to the neutral anatomical position. This will assist in maintaining core temperature control while awaiting transport. See Figure 3.3.

MOVING A VICTIM

If the site of the injury is hazardous, you'll need to get the victim (and you) away from it as quickly as possible. You may also need to move the injured person if he's incapable of walking out on his own, either to carry him out or get him to a rescue vehicle. Your key goal here is to be fast, efficient, and above all, not to further injure the patient. It's also a situation in which we can't emphasize enough the importance of remaining calm. It's possible to hurry without seeming hurried. See "Moving Techniques" later in this chapter for specifics on how to move an injured person. If hazardous conditions prevail, you're going to have to very quickly make a decision about whether to move the person—probably before you've even examined him. The methods we'll discuss here are easily mastered ways of accomplishing this.

MOVING TECHNIQUES

The following techniques are some of the most common methods of moving an injured person out of harm's way.

The Clothes Drag

The great advantage of this technique is that it isn't going to wear you out. The one thing it does need is a clear path between the victim's body and your destination. Clearly you can't have the patient bumping over rocks and sticks while being moved.

Pull the victim by his collar, hauling him in the direction you want. You can do a modified version of this technique, called the blanket roll, by gently maneuvering the patient onto a blanket and then dragging the blanket. See Figure 3.4.

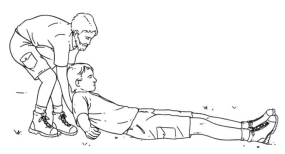

Figure 3.4. The clothes drag

One-Person Walk Assist

If the victim is alert and can move on her feet, put one of her arms behind your neck and hold her wrist. With your other hand around her waist, you can guide her to safety. See Figure 3.5.

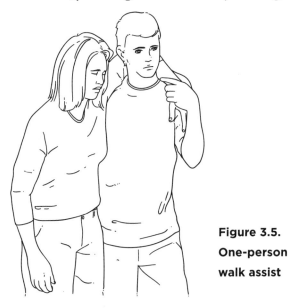

**Figure 3.5.
One-person
walk assist**

The Front Cradle

If the victim is small—especially if she is a child—use this technique to get her out. Keep in mind that it will wear you out quicker than some other techniques. The patient slips her arm around the back of the rescuer's neck while the rescuer lifts the patient under the lap, carrying her to the desired safe spot. See Figure 3.6.

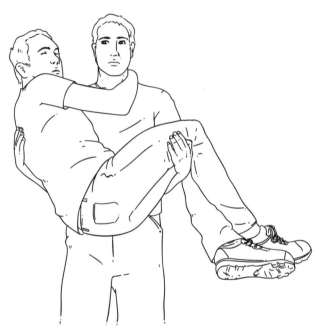

Figure 3.6. The front cradle

HELICOPTER EVACUATION AND SIGNALING

In certain emergencies, rescuers may need to pull the victim out by helicopter. In such cases, it's your responsibility to let them know where you are. Find the highest point close to where you are, and kindle a fire. Put on plenty of green stuff; that will both create white smoke and keep the fire under control. You can burn rubber and plastic if you want to create black smoke.

Take all the usual precautions when building and tending the fire. An out-of-control signal fire can do a lot of damage and could endanger your lives if it starts a forest fire.

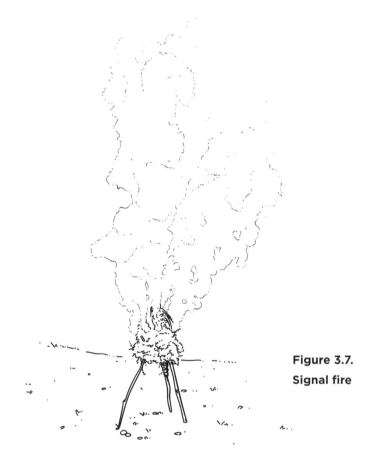

Figure 3.7.
Signal fire

Lighting a signal fire is the same as any other fire—just think bigger. Have multiple sure-fire ignition points in the fire lay as well as all the fuel and signal-type additives, such as green branches or pine bows, standing by. The main thing to remember with signal fires is to create an updraft to raise the smoke plume—so oxygen at the base is imperative. You may also consider a smoke generator, which is a fire shelf built on a tripod of sticks to allow maximum updraft for the fire.

First, construct a tripod with three green wood poles approximately 2" in diameter. Then add a shelf approximately one-third of the way up the legs. This will allow the oxygen to flow freely from the bottom and create a lot of smoke quickly. Once the fire lay is built on the shelf, the remaining upper frame can be stuffed with smoke-generating materials; have more standing by. See Figure 3.7.

Sometimes it's possible to create a visual call for help—marking it out in stones, for example. If you can mark out an SOS followed by a vertical line, observers will know you have an emergency that includes a serious injury. If you spot someone searching for you (from a helicopter, for example), raise both your arms in the air. This is the internationally recognized call for help. If you lie on the ground with your arms over your head, you're signaling that you or someone with you is injured. The hallmarks of signaling are contact and movement. For example, waving lit torches for circling aircraft or lighting three fires in a straight line will attract a lot of attention.

Don't let the signal fire go out; you don't know how long it's going to take for someone to notice it. If you need to sleep, get wood or other burnable materials to keep it going.

BUSHCRAFT TIP

A helicopter needs an area approximately 100′ × 100′ to land safely. If you can find such an area near where you are, the pilot will be able to identify this cleared area from his craft.

CARING FOR UNRESPONSIVE INJURED OR ILL PEOPLE

If the unresponsive person is a member of your group, think about what you know about his or her medical history and ask other group members for any information they have. If you don't know him, ask his friends or anyone else at the scene if they know something about what happened. If you're alone or if no one saw what occurred, it's going to be up to you to figure it out.

- For your own safety and that of the patient and others, make sure that the area is clear of any dangers.
- Apply BSI (body substance isolation).
- See if the victim has any medical bracelets or medallions. Check his wallet for anything that might indicate a chronic medical problem.
- Perform an exam along the lines of what we discussed earlier. Check his vital signs, responsiveness, and ABCs. Look for signs of a seizure (irregular heartbeat, bitten tongue, spasming muscles). If the ground around him is disturbed, it may be because he thrashed about.
- First care for the ABCs and any specific injuries identified during the physical exam.
- If the patient has vomited, move him into a recovery position unless you suspect an injury to the neck or spine. If he has not vomited, continue to maintain his ABCs until you can move him into a recovery position.
- Maintain body core temperature by wrapping the injured person with a blanket and protecting him from the elements.
- Turn him to the other side, again in a recovery position, every two hours to inhibit blood from pooling internally, which may cause bruising.
- Evacuate him as soon as possible.

If you're going to take care of someone who's unresponsive and you anticipate that it may take several days before either rescuers reach you or he becomes responsive, your priorities are shelter and warmth. This may require survival skills discussed in Chapter 2.

CARING FOR RESPONSIVE INJURED AND ILL PEOPLE

When a patient is alert and responsive, he will likely be capable of assisting in his own care, so ask him to help. For example, he can hold dressings in place while you bandage. Keep him engaged in his well-being and monitor for changes in vitals every fifteen minutes until EMS arrives.

Should the injured person only be responsive to verbal or painful stimuli, treat for shock by maintaining his core temperature, keep talking to him and giving psychological support (this encourages him to fight to be awake), and maintain ABCs. If he has vomited, move him into a recovery position unless injuries prevent such movement. Continue to monitor vitals every five minutes until EMS arrives.

TIPS AND TRICKS

- Heat up your water bottle and wrap it in a T-shirt to use as a heating pack for maintaining the core temperature of an ill or injured patient.
- Fill water bottles with cold water to use as cold packs for inflammation.
- Space blankets are reflective. Frames built for them can turn them into large signal mirrors to flash SOS.

— Chapter 4 —

TREATMENT OF BLEEDING AND WOUNDS

"So fragile—the human body. Just one prick and it will draw blood. Just one bullet and the bleeding never stops."

—Tiana Dalichov

Some of the most common outdoor injuries are cuts, scrapes, and puncture wounds. Often these are minor injuries but sometimes they are not. Even if a cut seems minor it can become infected if left untreated and lead to sepsis, a life-threatening illness.

STOP THE BLEEDING

The main goal in treating any bleeding injury is to stop the bleeding. To do this, apply direct pressure. Don't place your bare hands directly on a cut or wound. Use gloves or another impermeable barrier to protect yourself. See Figure 4.1.

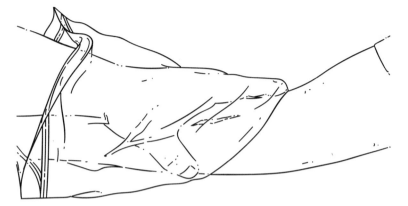

Figure 4.1. Direct pressure applied using a freezer bag

BUSHCRAFT TIP

It's quite possible that you won't have nitrile gloves with you. In that case, you need some nonabsorbent material to keep your skin and the blood apart. If you have any plastic bags (grocery, sandwich, etc.), those can do the job. So can a plastic trash bag or a Mylar blanket. If the injured party is known to you and you're reasonably sure he doesn't have a condition that could be transferred to you through blood, you can forego using gloves or a substitute.

DIRECT PRESSURE

If your patient has injured her arm or leg, raise the limb so it's above the heart. This will help slow the bleeding and make your job easier. Press down on the area and maintain that pressure for five to ten minutes. After ten minutes, if the patient is still bleeding, spread the pressure over a wider area and maintain it for another ten minutes.

If the patient has lost a lot of blood, she may go into shock, indicated by rapid breathing and pulse and possibly loss of consciousness. In these circumstances, you should keep her warm and, if she's awake, talk calmly to her to try to relieve her stress.

WOUND CLEANING AND BANDAGING

After you've stopped the bleeding, you will need to clean and protect the injured area. If the wound is very large or very deep, stop the bleeding but don't try to clean it. Seek medical attention immediately. When possible, allow the injured person to do the cleaning himself, as he will be able to adjust what he's doing to the amount of pain he's in.

Remove any obvious debris by brushing it away with a clean cloth or by using a pair of sterilized tweezers or a blunt-ended needle to pluck it out (in a pinch, heat tweezers/needle with a lighter to clean it; allow it to cool before using). If the material is deeply embedded, do not try to remove it but instead seek immediate medical help.

Once you have brushed away or otherwise removed obvious debris, flood the area with a large amount of clean water to flush away any remaining dirt or debris (see "Cleaning the Wound" later in this chapter for more information). Cool water will probably feel more comfortable than warm or hot water. Use soap to wash around the wounded area but don't try to dig into the wound itself (be careful when cleaning a wound near an eye so that soap does not get into the eye). The cleaning process may cause the wound to start bleeding again. If this happens, apply direct pressure to stop the bleeding.

Once the wound has been cleaned, protect it with a bandage and be sure to change the bandage at least once a day, or until professional medical help is obtained (then follow the medical professional's advice). When possible, use nonstick bandages and dressings so that removing them does not cause the wound to start bleeding again.

CLEANING THE WOUND

The best way to clean a wound is by irrigation—that is, running a forceful stream of water over it. A syringe is helpful for doing this, and if you have room in your pack, take along a 20 cc syringe. If you don't have one, cut a hole in a plastic bag and use that. If the wound is deep, disinfect some water and hold it 6–8" above the patient, then pour it onto the injury. Be careful not to let any of the blood spatter on you.

USING DISINFECTANTS AND OINTMENTS

Cleaning a wound with soap and water is the best way to prevent infection. People often think using disinfectants such as rubbing alcohol, peroxide, or iodine can help clean the wound and speed up healing, but these chemicals are too harsh to use on damaged tissues and can actually slow down the healing process. You can use disinfectants on the skin around a wound to help keep it clean but don't use them on the wound itself.

If you don't have any commercial antibiotics for treating shallow cuts, use pine sap. You can easily gather it, and it will protect the wound from infection.

CLOSING THE WOUND

Make some butterfly bandages from a roll of Gorilla Tape. You can use them to hold the edges of the wound together. See Figure 4.2.

If you can't get a wound to close with tape or butterfly bandages, place sterile dressings in the wound to keep it clean and protected and then cover it with a bandage. Change the dressings and the bandage itself at least once a day, until you can obtain help from a medical professional. Closing a wound is a way to help the tissue repair itself and to reduce the likelihood of infection but a wound doesn't have to be sutured right away—sutures can still be placed by a medical professional several days after an injury has occurred.

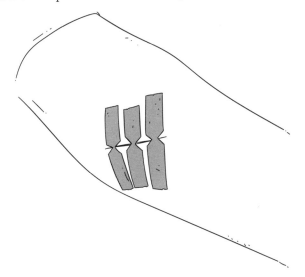

Figure 4.2. Butterfly bandages made from Gorilla Tape

LIMB FUNCTION

Sometimes a wound can injure tendons, ligaments, or even bones. For example, if someone in your party cuts his hand and can't move his fingers, it's probable that he severed a tendon. To determine how serious an injury is, you'll need to evaluate limb function. If an injury to the arm or hand has occurred, first check for the ability to move the hand and/or fingers. If the injured person can move them, check them for grip strength, which should be firm but not tight. If your patient has injured his leg or foot, place a hand on the bottom of his foot and ask him to press down. Then make the opposite test: put your hand over his foot and have him try to pull it up. This will tell you whether the blood is flowing as it should, how much strength there is in the limb, and whether the patient is experiencing pain in any kind of movement of his foot.

If a wound has injured a tendon, ligament, or bone, splint the affected limb to keep it immobile and protect the area. Although immediate professional medical care is desirable, tendon and other damage may be repaired even days after an injury.

CREATING AND APPLYING BANDAGES AND DRESSINGS

There's a difference between a dressing and a bandage. A dressing is placed directly on the wound, while a bandage holds it in place. You can make an effective dressing out of a piece of clean cloth. Double it over and hold it with a piece of Gorilla Tape. See Figure 4.3.

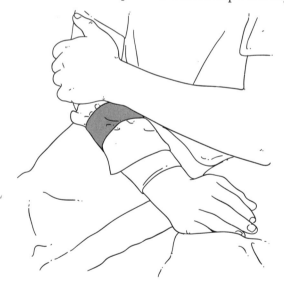

Figure 4.3. Dressing with Gorilla Tape bandage

The main thing in applying a dressing is to be as clean as possible so as to avoid infection. To that end, wash your hands. If the cloth is sterile, that's great, but if it's not, you're going to have to use it anyway. Find the clean part of it and use it. If time permits, boil it and let it dry before applying. Place the dressing material on the wound. If it's a large wound, you may need to wrap the dressing around the wound. Maintain even tension to ensure that circulation is not cut off. Then secure the dressing by tying it, using tape, or with whatever improvised item you can find. For the wilderness first-aider, do what works!

As a wound scabs over and begins to heal, it will probably cause the dressing to stick a bit. Not only can this be painful when it's time to change the dressing, but you need to be careful not to reopen the wound. You can get the dressing off by wiping around the stuck area with a damp cloth. As in all things in this book, be gentle and mindful of your patient's discomfort.

BUSHCRAFT TIP

As far as bandages in the wild go, you've got a lot of options. You can use gauze, Gorilla Tape, or tear strips of cloth from a piece of clothing.

NO-PRESSURE BANDAGING

You may need to dress and bandage a wound that has an open fracture (the bone is sticking out) or with embedded debris that cannot be immediately removed (such as glass or gravel that is not on the surface). In these cases, you will need to apply a no-pressure bandage so as not to cause the injured person additional pain. Use your bandaging material for this. Twist the bandaging material to create a rope-like effect. Shape this into a circle and place the center of the circle over the area you're trying to protect. Then gently secure the material in place.

SIGNS OF INCORRECT BANDAGING

If you have applied a bandage correctly, the bleeding should be stopped (or slowed) and the wound protected. If you've applied the bandage too tightly, it can restrict circulation and cause tissue damage. If there is a blue tinge in the nail beds, a feeling of coldness, or an inability to move the hand or foot below the bandaged wound, it is a sign of a too-tight bandage. So is pale skin around the bandage, a tingling feeling or loss of sensation near the bandaged area, or pain around the bandaged area that isn't because of the wound. If any of these things occur, it's best to rebandage the wound.

PRACTICAL SCENARIO

Earlier today, you gashed yourself with a knife while preparing a nice, hot campfire meal. You cleaned and bandaged it, using a good amount of pressure because the wound kept wanting to bleed. Now your hand feels a little cold and it's tingling. It's too dark to tell if it has changed color. What should you do?

ANSWER

A cold sensation and tingling are signs you've bandaged your cut too tightly. If you could see it better, you'd probably notice your fingernail beds were turning a little blue and your skin had turned paler. Remove the bandage and try again.

USING TOURNIQUETS

A tourniquet is a bandage or other device that compresses a limb and its blood vessels in order to reduce blood flow. See Figure 4.4.

The use of a tourniquet is a last resort and in fact is rarely needed. Improper application of a tourniquet may cause permanent damage to the tissues of the affected limb, leading to dire consequences such as amputation. As we talked about earlier, you can use direct pressure, elevation of the limb, and pressure points to control external bleeding without the need of a tourniquet. However, sometimes you don't have a choice: if the patient is continuing to lose blood, you should use a tourniquet.

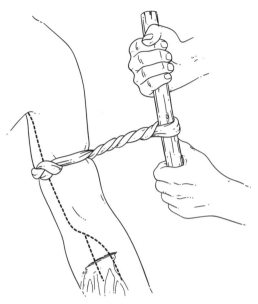

Figure 4.4. Example of a tourniquet

APPLYING A TOURNIQUET

Fashioning and applying a tourniquet isn't difficult as long as you keep a clear head and follow these steps.

1. Placement of the tourniquet is important. You want to place it 2" above the injury. In case that puts you on a joint, go 2" above the joint. Wrap the area with the tourniquet material. If you aren't using a professionally manufactured tourniquet, be careful with the one you've fashioned. The tourniquet should be approximately 2" wide and a few layers thick. Under no circumstances use rope or wire; they can further injure your patient. Belts aren't generally flexible enough to tie tightly. It's better to use a strip of cloth, a pack strap, a plastic drum liner, or something else that can be rolled up and tied.

2. Start tightening the tourniquet. When you see the bleeding stop, stop tightening. Leave it on until it's taken off by a medical

professional, since you don't want to loosen clots. These can get into the bloodstream and cause considerable damage.

3. If the patient is being evacuated and you're not going with him, pin a note to his clothing that will tell the doctor you've applied a tourniquet. It is best practice to place a TK (*TK* means "tourniquet") on the patient's forehead. Be sure to say when you put on the tourniquet.

PREVENTING AND IDENTIFYING INFECTION

Because of the way your body's infection-fighting white blood cells work, redness, heat, and tenderness in the area around an injury are the first signs that an infection is occurring. In the event of an infection, the lymphatic system kicks into high gear, carrying away unwanted stuff in your body. For this reason, red streaks may appear on the skin, pointing toward the heart. The patient's body temperature will increase—in other words, a fever—since some bacteria are negatively affected by heat.

An infection that starts to spread (indicated by the signs we just discussed) presents a serious danger to the patient. To treat it, you will want to draw bacteria from the wound in the form of pus. Soak a cloth in hot water and place it over the injury. If you don't have antibacterial medicine in your first-aid kit look for natural means to halt the infection. Find some tulip poplar leaves and put them in a bandanna, which you then put over the wound.

Any infection that lasts more than twelve hours is going to do sufficient damage to the patient that he'll require a hospital stay to fully recover. That being the case, your priority should be making and executing plans for an evacuation. This is especially important because it's unlikely that a person with a fever and spreading infection can walk out on his own. At the same time, you want to keep everyone else in the group safe. If the patient's skin is covered with boils or other symptoms, keep the rest of the party away from him.

Hot soaks can cause the wound to reopen. That's not a cause for alarm, since it means the wound is draining pus and other harmful substances. Don't make the hot soaks too hot, but make them as hot as is tolerable.

Once the wound has drained, prepare a new dressing. Twice a day, reopen the wound, drain it, and re-dress it.

SPECIAL WOUNDS

Certain types of bleeding injuries require care beyond merely stopping the bleeding and cleaning and bandaging the wound. These special wounds require special care.

SUCKING CHEST WOUNDS

Sucking chest wounds are a special category of injury in which something has penetrated the chest wall. If the hole is a small one, the body itself will seal it (although this is still a serious injury). If the hole is too big for the body to self-repair, though, this is a sucking chest wound. A small wound such as one from a thorn can self-seal when the object is removed, essentially allowing the surrounding material to return to its proper position. In the event of a large penetrating object—such as impalement by an arrow or a broken-off tree limb—the hole is so large that when the victim breathes and her chest expands, she also sucks in air through the hole. If the injury isn't properly treated, this can collapse the lung.

It's not sufficient to put a dressing and a bandage over the injury. This is a wound you have to treat in a special manner: you have to make a valve.

From some nonstick material—for example, a piece of plastic—cut a piece three to four times bigger than the hole. Using Gorilla Tape, seal three of the four sides of the bandage and leave one side open. This creates what's called a flutter valve. An inhale will pull the bandage down against the hole and prevent air from entering it. An exhale will push the patch away from the hole temporarily.

FLAIL CHEST

Flail chest is a serious condition that results from multiple fractures of the rib cage caused by blunt force trauma; this is common in the wilderness due to falls from tree stands, ATV accidents, and stumbles while hiking. What's happened here is that some of the ribs have been separated from the chest wall. When the victim breathes out, these ribs will push against the skin, creating a bulge, which will disappear when he breathes in. The patient will have trouble breathing and, because broken ribs are extremely painful, probably express great distress.

Place a folded blanket or some other soft padding over the area. Be very gentle while doing this; after all, you're dealing with broken bones. This is a case where you should try to evacuate the patient swiftly so trained medical professionals can deal with the situation.

GUNSHOT WOUNDS

Since outdoorsmen are often hunters, accidental gunshot wounds sometimes occur. A single bullet can cause multiple internal and external injuries. Treatments are very limited in remote locations, but the following options will be useful for four types of GSWs (gunshot wounds).

SUPERFICIAL GSW

Treat superficial wounds as you would any other puncture wound. Apply pressure, dress the wound, and apply a pressure bandage. Keep in mind that a GSW may have caused damage in the tissue surrounding the actual entry point. Bullets rarely follow a straight line when they enter the body and the bullet may have ricocheted or bounced off a bone, creating fragments, so do a careful assessment of the injured person to be certain you understand the full extent of the injury.

GSW TO THE ARM OR LEG

Apply direct pressure and elevate the wound immediately followed by a pressure bandage. If it's still bleeding, apply pressure to a pressure point then after thirty minutes if nothing has slowed, apply a tourniquet. The upper thigh is the site of the femoral artery. If the GSW is in that part of the body, apply a tourniquet immediately. Think about shattered bone fragments and internal injuries: if the area swells rapidly, that's a sign of internal bleeding. If bones appear broken, you'll need to immobilize the limb once bleeding is controlled.

GSW TO THE ABDOMEN

Think about protecting the internal organs. Bullet damage to the hollow organs of the abdomen can lead to a number of harmful conditions including severe internal bleeding. If you discover protruding intestines, place a moist, sterile dressing on top of the wound (to protect the organs). If the intestines are damaged or torn open, immediate medical care is required. If the injured person does not bleed out first, he may likely die due to severe bacterial infection that will ensue. Make certain the injured person does not eat or drink anything until the pain lets up, then he should only sip clear fluids for a day or two after. Rehydration via IV fluids will likely be required once the injured person is in a hospital setting.

GSW TO THE CHEST

Spinal injuries and sucking air into the chest are two major concerns with a GSW to the chest. If the wound is open, creating a sucking chest wound, treat it as such by applying an occlusive dressing so that a lung doesn't collapse. If you suspect spinal injury, do not move the injured person as fragmented bone or bullet particles could make the spinal condition and internal bleeding worsen. If the heart, lungs, or a major blood vessel is damaged, there's nothing you can do in a remote area without proper expert medical care.

BUSHCRAFT TIP

In nearly all cases you should not attempt to remove an implanted bullet while in the field. Most are nearly impossible to locate, and some may actually be aiding in the prevention of worsening bleeding once lodged.

KNIFE AND AXE INJURIES

Most knife and axe injuries in the wilderness are superficial and can easily be controlled with direct pressure, elevation, and proper dressing and bandaging without the need for sutures or ointments.

For more serious wounds such as stabbings and deep lacerations, stopping the blood loss is of immediate importance. You can best accomplish this by using clotting agents, tampons, scarves, shirts, or other sterile absorbents.

Many plants contain tannins. These are a drying as well as constricting agent, and they work well in masticated or powdered form to help stop bleeding. Depending on the type of wound you may use different types of plants as aid if you have nothing else. Yarrow flower tops and leaves work well for deep gashes, and common goldenrod works well on superficial bleeding. Many plants are absorbent to some extent and can be used directly for bandages or as a medium between layers to absorb blood. Mullein has large, broad, soft leaves that will work as standalone gauze, while you can use things such as cattail fluff as a batting material to help soak up blood in between dressings. See Chapter 16 for more information on using plants to help heal injuries and illnesses sustained in the wild.

As a general rule, wounds that remain closed on their own do not require sutures; you can clean them and keep them closed with butterfly bandages or duct tape. Deeper wounds that remain open on their own, however, should not be sutured in the field due to the likelihood of bacterial infection and the possibility of them constantly opening back up. So keep those types of wounds clean and covered with dressings and bandages.

When medical help is less than an hour away, you can get away with a lot more in wound care. Wash it out with whatever clean water you have and slap a bandage on it, and you're pretty much good to go.

SELF-AID

What if you're at camp, all alone, a day away from any sort of help and you chop into your inner thigh and cut your femoral artery? You could likely bleed out in as little as two minutes if you don't act fast. If you are alone and ill prepared, you're in trouble. Even if you have someone there to assist, you could still bleed out if you don't act quickly.

The quickest solution is to apply a tourniquet to stop the bleeding. Then you need to clean the wound carefully. Wash it with clean water and soap.

After you clean your life-threatening wound, you need to somehow clot the blood. Celox is the best clotting agent currently available, but another option that is doable so long as you do not have a shellfish allergy is sterile powdered shellfish carapace (exoskeletons of crabs, lobster, shrimp), which is the base of many common clotting agents such as Celox. Or, use wood ash to pack the wound.

Once bleeding is controlled, lie down, elevate the injury, and try and relax. Await help and if possible, scoot yourself into a safer place to shelter until that help arrives.

TIPS AND TRICKS

- Use a credit card or driver's license as a "dressing" to help stop bleeding and protect a wound.
- Sterilize cloth in the wilderness by boiling it and laying it out in direct sunlight to dry.
- You can create simple bandages using 1"-wide duct tape and a small square of cotton T-shirt.
- You can make a fomentation to treat local swelling from abrasions by soaking a piece of cotton material in an infusion of anti-inflammatory herbs such as plantain or jewelweed. See Chapter 16 for more on fomentations and infusions.
- Large mullein leaves make a fine emergency replacement for feminine pads if the need arises.

— Chapter 5 —

BLISTERS
AND BURNS

"Pain is inevitable. Suffering is optional."

—ORIGIN UNKNOWN

Blisters and burns are common injuries for those exploring the great outdoors. Often these are minor but sometimes they can be major; in any case they can take the fun out of the experience, so learning how to treat (and prevent!) them is crucial.

PREVENTING AND TREATING BLISTERS

At some time in our lives, practically all of us have experienced the pain and annoyance of blisters. Their cause is the rubbing of skin, which causes the outer layer to tear away from the secondary layer. In between the two layers, fluid accumulates, pushing the outer layer into a bulge.

We have found that the best socks for long-term wilderness use are made of wool. Wool socks in all their variants such as alpaca, merino, and various blends not only have a natural ability to repel odor and water, but they keep most of their insulating value even when wet. For avid hikers, we also recommend wearing sock liners such as polyblend compression socks, which aid in wicking away moisture while preventing the main sock from rubbing against the skin.

Obviously, the key to avoiding blisters on your feet is to reduce the friction on them. You can use one of these methods:

- Fit boots properly.
- Put padding in your boots that protect your feet from places they're likely to chafe.
- Wear two pairs of socks to reduce sliding.
- Tape your feet with moleskin or surgical tape. If you have any pre-existing sores on your feet, make sure they're covered and padded.
- Going downhill increases the tendency of your feet to slide around in their boots. Make sure that before you start down a slope, your boots are tightened.

SELF-AID

Whatever kind of boots you buy, the most important thing is that they fit properly. The longer you wear leather boots, the better they'll fit as the leather gradually assumes the shape of your feet. Plastic boots don't have this quality, so make sure when you buy them that they're an optimal fit. Above all, buy boots you feel comfortable in. Ill-fitting boots can make a simple walk in the woods a nightmare. In wet weather, coat your feet with petroleum jelly before putting on socks not only to soothe the effects of all-day wet feet but also to lessen the chances of blisters caused by the friction of wet socks.

Blisters on your hands can occur because of repetitive motions with tools, such as digging with a shovel or performing extended carving tasks with your knife.

To prevent blisters on your hands:

- If you feel a hot spot develop, address it by covering the affected area with duct tape, moleskin, or another type of dressing.
- Wear gloves that fit well when using tools, especially for repetitive-motion tasks.
- Working with tools often will help to build calluses on the hands, preventing hot spots. If you only use tools occasionally and all of a sudden have to do heavy work or work for an extended period, watch for hot spots and treat as discussed previously.
- Another thing that commonly causes blisters, especially from wood-handled tools, is the lacquer coating placed on many tools by the manufacturer; this coating causes friction and should be sanded to remove it. Then the handle should be oiled with a linseed oil to protect it.
- Excessive heat and cold can also cause blisters. Protect yourself from the elements appropriately. See Chapter 13 for more information on treating frostbite and sunburn.
- Contact dermatitis can cause blistering. See Chapter 15 for more information on preventing and treating plant-induced dermatitis.
- Bug bites can also cause blisters, so using an insect repellent can help. If a blister becomes itchy, apply a small amount of hydrocortisone to the affected area. See Chapter 14 for additional information on insect bites.
- Blisters can be a sign of chickenpox or shingles, so if you have additional symptoms, such as a fever or chills, seek medical advice. Also, blisters around the eyes and the genitals are a particular cause of concern and deserve medical attention.

BUSHCRAFT TIP

As with any wound, blisters can become infected, so watch out for signs of infection—warmth and redness around the affected area, red streaks leading from the affected area, greenish pus coming from the blister (instead of watery clear fluid). Seek medical help if you suspect an infection.

In treating blisters, take the following steps:

- Sterilize the blade of your knife, or a needle if you have one. You can use rubbing alcohol to do this.
- Pierce and drain the blister.
- Use decontaminated water to flush out the blister.
- Dry it and put a dressing and bandage on it.
- If the blister is large, don't pierce it; instead make a doughnut dressing, place it around the blister, and secure it in place with a bandage.
- If necessary, use Super Glue or pine sap to close the wound.

FOOT ROT/TRENCH FOOT

Trench foot was a common problem faced by soldiers in World War I. Sometimes called foot rot or immersion foot, it is a tissue injury to your feet when they've been cold and wet for too long. If you have trench foot, your feet will feel numb at first—not too serious, you say. However, if you don't address it at this early stage, and especially if you develop blisters on your feet, matters can get much worse; your feet can swell, you'll lose sensation, and you'll be in considerable pain. To prevent it, change your socks frequently and keep your feet clean, warm, and dry. Rub ashes from your fire on your feet. This is an effective prevention against trench foot, since it keeps your feet dry. See Figure 5.1.

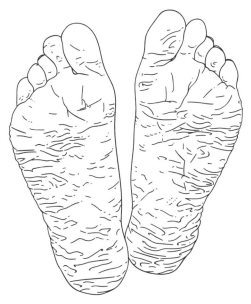

**Figure 5.1. Foot rot, also known as trench foot
and immersion foot**

SELF-AID

I (Jason) suffered from trench foot during one of the Pathfinder Scout classes. I observed good foot hygiene, changed socks often, and even changed boots, often cycling through three different pairs, rubber and hiker style. The class took place in rainy conditions with high humidity even when it was not raining. So when the sun was out, my feet would sweat, and when it rained, they just got wetter. Each night I'd warm them by the fire in the open air, but the condition really worsened when I got back home. The entire bottom of both feet became a blister, which had to be peeled off. After a couple of days of staying off my feet, I was able to walk around again, albeit in pain. When you think you have enough socks, bring more, especially if you're expecting inclement weather conditions.

BURNS IN THE WILD

A burn can range from a mild injury from touching a hot pan to a major trauma that occurs because your clothes catch on fire. Your immediate priority is to stop any burning that's still going on. If someone's clothes are on fire, roll her on the ground to put out the flames or use cold water. In the event someone scalds herself, get the pieces of clothing covering the scald off as soon as possible; they're trapping the heat next to the burn and making it worse.

If burned clothing sticks to the skin, don't try to remove it but instead reduce the heat with cool water.

Next you need to cool the burn itself. If water is available, use that. Of course it's best to use clean water, but this is a time-dependent emergency; use the cleanest water available. If you're not near a water source, use cool soil, wet leaves or moss, or other natural means to cool the wound. Before you place these on the wound, cover it with plastic.

If the burn is severe (10 percent of the body or more), don't try to cool the burn using water as this could lead to hypothermia. Instead, focus on dressing the burn and getting immediate help.

MOIST VERSUS DRY DRESSINGS

Generally speaking, burn protocol requires the application of dry dressings to be placed on burns. This is due to the fact that moist (wet) dressings can sap heat away from the body, putting the burned person at risk for hypothermia. Moist dressings, however, typically make the patient feel better and also reduce the need for pain medications. So, here are some guidelines:

- When treating superficial burns (first degree), leave them dry. These burns require the least intervention unless they are in a painful area such as the face, neck, or other sensitive area.
- In partial-thickness or full-thickness burn cases (second and third degree), you may apply moist dressings to soothe and manage

pain so long as they are not applied to more than 10 percent of the body. Your arm is about 9 percent of the surface area of your body, so keep that in mind as a handy reference. Anything more than this covered with a moist dressing could certainly lead to hypothermia because of the body's inability to regulate temperature.

APPLYING A MOIST DRESSING

To apply a moist dressing:

1. Clean the burned area as with any wound.
2. Dampen (do not soak) clean cloth dressings such as a bandanna, T-shirt, or gauze if you have them.
3. Apply the moist material to the affected area, making certain that the burn area is less than 10 percent of total body surface area; otherwise hypothermia may result.
4. Keep the dressing damp by using a secondary wet dressing to transfer moisture to the one on the burn; do not pour water onto the dressing.
5. Treat for shock by keeping the patient talking and maintaining core body temperature.

Try to relieve as much pain as a possible through proper wound care (appropriate burn dressing) and by keeping the injured person calm. You can offer ibuprofen or similar pain relievers. Certain plants can also help provide relief from pain—see Chapter 16 for more information.

Burns, especially severe ones, cause your body to lose fluid. To deal with this, administer electrolytes, although only at half strength. Don't let the injured person become dehydrated.

BURN CLASSIFICATION

Assessing the seriousness of a burn helps you determine how to treat it and whether you need to seek medical attention immediately.

- If the victim has been superficially burned, the skin in the area affected will be red. Press the center of the burned area; when you release the pressure, the skin will turn from white back to red again. While this kind of burn is certainly painful, it won't require a dressing. (Think of the last time you had a light sunburn to get an idea of what this kind of burn looks like.) Cool off the affected area with water or a cold compress such as a water-filled canteen until pain is alleviated.

- More severe burns, called partial-thickness burns, have penetrated several layers of skin. If you've experienced a severe sunburn in which your skin not only turned red but blistered, you've had a partial-thickness burn. Partial-thickness burns may be dressed with a dry dressing. More severe burns, such as those caused by fire, can be dressed with a moist dressing. (Remember not to use moist dressings on burns that cover 10 percent or more of the body.)

- The most severe burns are called full-thickness burns. Here the injury has penetrated all layers of the skin. Oddly, some areas of the burn may hurt less than more superficial burns. That's because nerve endings have been damaged. On the other hand, the area around the burn is likely to hurt quite a bit. A moist dressing will aid in reducing pain and will soothe the area more than a dry dressing. If immediate evacuation is not possible, a moist dressing is the best course of action so long as the affected area is no greater than 10 percent of the total body surface area.

WHEN TO SEEK MEDICAL HELP FOR BURNS

If the victim has been burned over more than 5 percent of his body, your immediate plan, after treating and dressing the wound, should be evacuation. This is due to the fact that treatment in remote locations for burns is severely limited. The skin is our strongest defense against various forms of infection, and once it's burned away, we're at a much greater risk of contracting an infection. If the patient is burned over 20 percent or more of his body, he should be evacuated. Full-thickness-burn patients should always be evacuated as quickly as possible. If the victim is showing other symptoms (e.g., shivering uncontrollably, delusions, vomiting), he should be evacuated as soon as possible, since there may well be other injuries caused by the burn.

PRACTICAL SCENARIO

While canoe camping in the Boundary Waters of Minnesota, one of your friends has a bit too many to drink at camp around the fire. He begins to get animated telling a story and trips, then falls headfirst into the fire. You and your other three buddies scramble to pull him out. Then what would you do?

ANSWER

This scenario is sadly quite common, and the injuries sustained are not always limited to burns. They may include blunt force trauma to the abdomen and head and even injuries to the face such as broken teeth.

The first course of action is to stop any burning. Put out any fire on the victim's clothing or hair. Then make certain the injured person's airway is not compromised by severe burns, blood, or swelling. Burns will be determined by how long he was in the fire and what he fell on or if he braced his fall.

If he fell in and rolled out as you pulled him—not staying in contact with the fire for very long—it is likely that he only suffered superficial burns. But if he was excessively drunk and everyone else moved at the pace of a stunned drunkard, too, he may have lain in the fire for a few moments and perhaps braced his fall with his hands, attempting to push himself up on the hot coals. In this case, more severe partial-thickness burns along with superficial burns would be expected along with burning or at least melted outer garments.

Cooling burned areas is next on the list, as this will not only alleviate his pain but also bring down swelling. Do this while another person in your group is preparing burn dressings. It's at this time you'll be able to get an idea of the severity of the burns and if immediate evacuation will be required. Once you get a handle on the severity of the burns, you can begin to dress them appropriately and if available, administer some basic pain medication such as ibuprofen or apply any available burn gels. If there is cell reception, a call to the ranger station or 911 is also a good idea; they will advise on possible evacuation details. More likely than not, you'll be paddling out to a certain point, and unless you're a navigation wiz, it's not a good idea to take this on in the middle of the night while partially inebriated. You'll reassess your patient every five to fifteen minutes depending on burn severity and await daylight to assist in evacuation to proper medical care.

TIPS AND TRICKS

- For major pain relief in the field, consider giving (or taking) 1,000 mg of acetaminophen with 800 mg of ibuprofen; it provides the equivalent relief of some popular narcotic medications. Do not take more than three times in one day and do not take over an extended period.
- Wool does not burn as readily as cotton or synthetic material, so it's an excellent choice for outer garments such as shirts and jackets.
- The slime contained in the shoots of cattail is akin to aloe vera; it works as a topical anesthetic as well as an anti-inflammatory and is great for minor burns, including sunburn.
- Reducing anxiety can aid in reducing pain, stress, and the severity of injuries by relieving muscle spasms.

Chapter 6

BONE AND JOINT INJURIES

"The success of Egyptian surgery in setting broken bones is very fully demonstrated in the large number of well-joined fractures found in the ancient skeletons."
—JAMES HENRY BREASTED

Bone and joint injuries are the most common types of injuries in the outdoors—and people have been successfully treating them for thousands of years. The majority of outdoor injuries occur as the result of a stumble or fall but bone and joint injuries can also occur through repetitive use (a stress fracture after an unusually long trek, for example) or improper physical conditioning before undertaking strenuous tasks. Such injuries are fairly common among weekend warriors—people who have desk jobs and sedentary lifestyles throughout the week and who then over-exert themselves during a weekend camping trip. Remember, if you haven't been on a hiking trip for ten years, you should build up to your grand adventure of hiking the Appalachian Trail from Maine to Georgia.

TREATING FRACTURES

Broken bones come in all shapes and sizes. The most serious kind of break is a fracture, in which the bone has been broken to the extent that the ends of the break have separated. There are two kinds of fractures: open and closed.

- **Open fracture.** The broken end of the bone has penetrated the skin from the inside and pushed through it.
- **Closed fracture.** The broken ends of the bone have separated but are still beneath the skin. In such a fracture, you may notice a bulge where one of the broken ends is pushing up against the skin but hasn't penetrated it. This is called tenting.

Both kinds of fractures are extremely serious, and if there is an open wound near a fracture, it offers an opportunity for bacteria to infect the body.

SELF-AID

Fractures are hard enough to treat if other people have them, doubly so if the victim is you. You're in a lot of pain, but the most important thing is to be calm so you can evaluate your injury. Address bleeding first as it will be difficult to treat the break if it is still bleeding freely. See Chapter 4 for more information on how to stop bleeding.

Once bleeding is addressed, examine the fracture itself. If it's closed with no bone end protruding through the skin, you may slowly reduce any misalignment of the bone by moving it back into a normal body position. Some breaks, such as an open fracture, may be too bad to allow this. When the bone ends come through the skin, leave it alone and clean and cover the exposed bone. Careful examination is required to have a fair understanding of what's possible.

We'll assume it's a simple closed fracture, so your objective is not to set the bone back into place, but to move it back into a normal, resting position. For example, if your forearm is bent at a 90° angle, cradling the arm and moving it back to a flatter position will ease discomfort and make splinting a little more manageable.

Once you've examined the fracture and if needed, reduced it, splint and immobilize the injured area. Again, in the case of a fractured forearm, you might use a folded emergency blanket to cradle under the arm to provide padding for a splint while you then place a stiff stick alongside it to be taped. This will immobilize the fracture, preventing unwanted motion to and fro. Then by tying a couple of bandannas together, you create a cravat or sling that will cradle your elbow and keep your arm close to your chest, again in an effort to minimize motion of the injured limb and protect it from unnecessary bumps during evacuation.

TREATING THE WOUND

As we said earlier, a wound near a fracture is a serious issue, and you should address it first. Do what's necessary to slow and stop the bleeding (pressure points, dressing, and bandage). Pressure here is tricky because of the fracture; rather than use direct pressure, employ pressure points, those pulse points between the injury and the heart that can be pressed to control bleeding.

Once you've controlled and halted the bleeding (or if the wound isn't bleeding much in the first place), clean the area with disinfected water and put a dressing and bandage on it. At this point you can address the fracture itself. Gently put a splint on it, being sensitive to the patient's pain. In some closed fractures, there will be no exterior open wound at all, so just take care not to aggravate any bruising as you treat the fracture.

PRESSURE POINTS

A pressure point is a place on the body where an artery can be pressed against a bone to slow bleeding. The quickest way to locate a pressure point is at the pulse point between the wound and the heart. Palpate (feel with the fingers) along a limb until you find a strong pulse and apply pressure at that point to reduce bleeding. Some of these points are found in the neck (carotid), at the end of the wrist, in the bend of the elbows, under the arm, and at the top of the thigh in the groin.

SPLINTING THE FRACTURE

A splint immobilizes the injured bone to keep it from further damage and to reduce pain. So anything you find that will get the job done is fine, so long as it does not pose any risk of further injury.

Treatment should not further injure the fractured area; protect open fractures and keep closed fractures closed. By definition, an open fracture creates a wound that can lead to infection all the way down to the bone marrow. Therefore, it's vitally important to keep open fractures clean, covered, and protected until you reach definitive medical care. Keep a closed fracture from becoming an open one by properly splinting and immobilizing the injury site. It would be a terrible thing for a broken bone to cut its way through tented skin during evacuation along a rough trail.

When you're splinting a fracture, it's very important to take bleeding into consideration, particularly the arteries, since a severed artery can cause the patient to bleed out. To guard against this, make padding and pack it around the splint wherever it seems loose.

Since the injured person should be evacuated as soon as possible, you'll be faced with the problem of moving him while creating as little movement as you can of the injured limb. The weather can present challenges; if you used metal for the splint, it will adjust its temperature to outside air, so if it's very cold, you'll need to wrap the splint in something to insulate it.

You can fashion a splint using the following pack items:

- Cargo tape
- Cordage
- Cutting tool
- Emergency blanket (this can also be fashioned into a sling)

For the splint itself, a sturdy branch or bough stripped of leaves and twigs will work splendidly.

Whatever natural material you use, do your best to keep dirt away from the wound itself and maintain a clean dressing. See Figures 6.1, 6.2, 6.3, and 6.4.

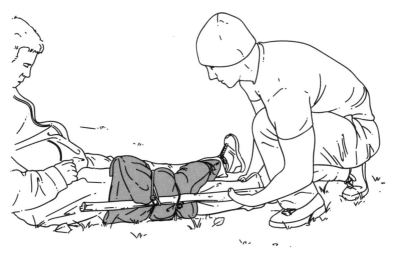

Figure 6.1. Leg splint (notice the padding around the joint)

After splinting the fracture, elevate the injured limb if possible to reduce swelling.

Figure 6.2. Arm splint, heavily padded and cord wrapped

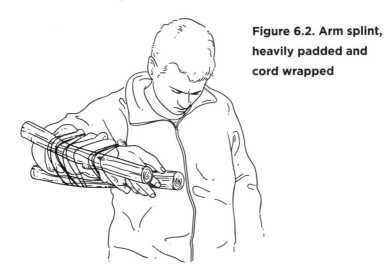

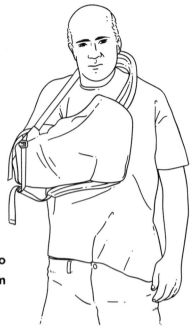

Figure 6.3. Backpack used to immobilize fractured arm

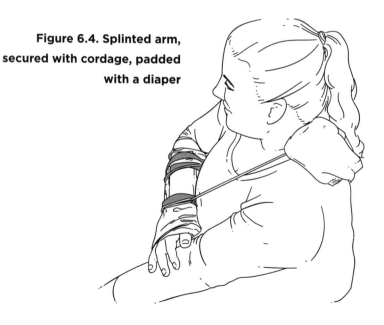

Figure 6.4. Splinted arm, secured with cordage, padded with a diaper

When treating a fractured limb, the injured person can assist you in wrapping, padding, and holding the limb to keep it from jostling around.

If the victim has injured her leg and is lying down, you can use a small-diameter stick to snake up a pant leg. Once upward pressure is applied to the stick, it serves as a crane. The pants serve as a cradle for the limb as you move it into position.

Another method is as follows: use both your hands to hold the joints and gently pull them apart. This will prevent the break from sagging while you splint it.

TRACTION SPLINTS

To treat fractured femurs (thigh bones), you'll need to make a traction splint. A traction splint, ideally, is a manufactured apparatus that will secure the upper and lower leg with a tension device at the foot. Wraps are placed around the ankle of the injured leg and then a screw is turned to provide tension on the wraps on the distal (lower) portion of the leg allowing it to lightly separate from the upper half, thereby reducing pain and the potential for the broken bone to rub against the other or cause injury to the femoral artery.

> **BUSHCRAFT TIP**
> Any thigh injury, including a fracture of the femur, is serious, since your thigh is the site of the femoral artery. Damage to this blood vessel can be fatal, because it will release a large amount of blood (if nothing else, this will probably cause the patient to go into shock).

It's very unlikely that you carried in a traction device. Fortunately they're easy to make, especially if you have ski poles or a walking stick. Splint the outside leg its entire length, going up to the armpit. Splint the inside leg to the groin. Now wrap the leg (which helps to hold the splints in place) and create a wrap for the ankle. Attach a cross stick to the bottom of the splints and attach one end of the ankle wrap. Use a twisting stick to increase tension on the bottom of the splint. See Figure 6.5.

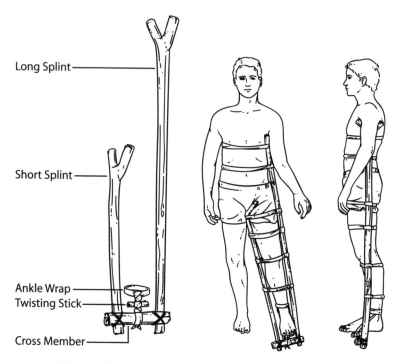

Long Splint

Short Splint

Ankle Wrap
Twisting Stick

Cross Member

Figure 6.5. Traction splint from wooden material

TREATING DISLOCATIONS

A dislocation is an injury to a joint that causes the bones of the joint to spread apart. You can see a dislocation because the joint will look wrong. The affected person will not be able to move the joint (or movement will be difficult and extremely painful). Any joint can become dislocated as a result of an injury.

Treat a dislocation much as you would a fracture. Stop bleeding, clean and dress the wounds, and splint the limb. If the dislocation has happened to a finger, kneecap, or shoulder, you can try to put the bone back in place. If the dislocation has happened to the hip, ankle, or elbow, get a professional medical person to treat it. Trying to force these joints to reduce may cause further injury.

> **SELF-AID**
>
> Self-reduction in the case of a dislocated joint is entirely possible, and the joint may go back into place with any attempted movement. You treat a dislocation as you would a closed fracture: control bleeding, splint the injury, and immobilize the area.

While pain will be relieved by reduction, there will still be residual soreness and stiffness, so acetaminophen or ibuprofen, if available, are acceptable for pain relief. A tea of willow bark would also be helpful as willow contains salicin, a naturally occurring aspirin. Just be certain you can properly identify the tree and understand how to use it correctly and only do so if you're without an allergy to aspirin.

CARING FOR SPRAINS, STRAINS, AND CRAMPS

Damage to the tissues of a joint caused by stretching or twisting results in a *sprain*. Such stretching or twisting often occurs when you fall or if you slip or make a misstep. The damage to the tissue causes swelling, which inhibits movement. Pain is another common symptom. Keep the RICE procedure in mind:

- Rest
- Ice
- Compression
- Elevation

Always give support to the injured limb by splinting or taping it.

Strains are pulled or torn muscles. Any type of unusual motion, like a fall or a sudden action, can cause the muscle to twist or move beyond its typical range, resulting in damage to the muscle fibers. To treat, apply the RICE procedure, and stretch gently.

Rest, compression, and elevation are fairly simple procedures, but ice is typically not available in the wilderness three seasons of the year. You can substitute a water bottle filled with cool water to be used as a cold pack or wrap strips of wet cotton loosely around the injured area and allow evaporation to cool the injury site.

Muscle cramps are unintended contractions in the muscle (that is, you're not deliberately using the muscle to perform a certain function). They occur because of some type of stress on the muscle. This stress could include holding it in one position for a long time or it could be the result of a muscle strain. Dehydration can also cause muscle cramps.

Stretching the cramping muscle can often make it feel better. You can also apply pressure to the area. Ice, if available, can often calm down a cramping muscle. For cramping caused by dehydration, give plenty of water.

ANKLE INJURIES

Ankle injuries are common in the outdoors. Ankle sprains can range from mild to severe in nature. Symptoms are sudden pain, swelling, bruising, and an inability to walk. If the sprain is mild, you may only experience some tenderness when touching it and may not have any, or very little, swelling. On the other hand, in severe cases, the swelling may be substantial and the pain intolerable; putting weight on the foot may be next to impossible.

Similarly to ankle sprains, ankle fractures are a common type of injury. However, unlike ankle sprains, a broken ankle always requires medical attention. With the symptoms so similar, how can you tell a broken or sprained ankle apart? Well, there are a few distinguishing signs to keep in mind.

First, ask the person to try to recall if there was a sound when she was injured. A "cracking" noise may be a sign that the ankle is broken while sprains are often associated with a "popping" sound.

Second, check if the ankle, in addition to being swollen, appears deformed or crooked as this may be a sign of a fracture. Third, the presence of numbness is indicative of a fracture. Moreover, if the person cannot move the ankle joint at all, is in extreme pain, and cannot put any weight at all on the ankle, it is likely that it is broken.

PRACTICAL SCENARIO

Let's say you're hiking along the Appalachian Trail and you come across a fellow hiker who is sitting and rubbing at his ankle in obvious distress. How can you help this person? How can you tell if the injury is just a sprain or a more serious matter, such as a fracture?

ANSWER

As you approach, announcing yourself and how you're trained in first aid, you do a quick scene survey to determine the MOI (mechanism of injury). Once you determine the scene is safe, you ask what happened. The hiker replies, "I tripped over a root and fell, but my foot was caught under the root and it popped as I hit the ground. It really hurts." You ask if there is pain anywhere else and as you look at him you see no obvious blood or other injuries. He replies that the ankle is all that hurts. So, you begin to asses the injured limb.

This patient reports a "popping" sound and you can see the ankle is severely swollen. So you would adhere to the RICE protocol in an effort to reduce localized pain and swelling. After he has calmed down and gotten a handle on the pain, you must consider evacuation, depending on how far you are from a roadway or town. This may dictate how you proceed. For this case, you decide to walk to the nearest shelter with the injured person because the shelter is near and the terrain is not rough. From there you will be able to get further help. You pull out your extra boots and reinforce your compression wrap with a tightly tied boot on the injured person's foot and offer him some over-the-counter pain medicine; then, you begin your journey to the shelter where you will re-evaluate the injury and rescue plan.

TIPS AND TRICKS

- Should you suffer from a broken bone, avoid carbonated soft drinks as their phosphorus content can weaken the healing process. Also avoid caffeine, which binds to important calcium molecules, preventing bones from absorbing what they need.
- Think about the boots you wear when traveling in the woods. In a hunting scenario, it is best to wear neoprene and rubber-type pull-on boots. These can easily be pulled on and off with only one hand and fit better over a swollen ankle if necessary.
- A strip of T-shirt cut from around the bottom into a strip about 6" wide makes a great emergency elastic bandage (like an Ace bandage).
- Practice skills such as fire building with your nondominant hand. Most of us will catch our fall with the dominant hand, and injuries occur most commonly during a fall or trip. Knowing how to use your other hand for essential tasks can keep an injury from turning into a disaster.

— Chapter 7 —

CIRCULATORY ISSUES

"All truly great thoughts are conceived while walking."
—Friedrich Nietzsche

Circulatory issues are those that relate to the heart, blood, and blood vessels. Sometimes they can be related to an illness, either chronic (such as peripheral artery disease) or acute (such as a heart attack), or they may result from another injury (as in the case of shock). For managing chronic illnesses while still enjoying the great outdoors, see Chapter 12.

IDENTIFYING AND TREATING SHOCK

Circulatory shock (sometimes called hypoperfusion or just "shock") results when an inadequate amount of blood is getting to tissue. It can be caused by loss of blood or anything else that creates dangerously low blood pressure. Our organs depend on blood to carry nutrients, oxygen, and other materials to them; when they don't get enough blood, they stop functioning. Although there are a number of different kinds of shock, in wilderness first aid we are primarily concerned with a few of the most common types. If left untreated, shock can lead to death.

TYPES OF SHOCK

Hypovolemic shock refers to a condition in which the amount of blood in the victim's body has decreased past a dangerous point. It can be caused by excessive bleeding, particularly from a severed artery. (This kind of shock is also called *hemorrhagic* shock.) Treatment is to stop the bleeding and dress and bandage the wound.

You can also experience hypovolemic shock if your body is dehydrated and the body starts sending water instead of blood. It can also be the result of severe burns (remember, we said earlier that one symptom of a severe burn can be dehydration). In both cases, increasing fluid consumption can help prevent the problem. Look for: rapid, weak pulse; low blood pressure; change in mental status; cool, clammy skin; and an increased respiratory rate. If the patient displays these, she may be in shock.

SELF-AID

The best way to avoid any health problems in the wild is to anticipate them and prevent them before they occur. Proper hydration in the field is an example. A typical 200-pound male needs approximately 64 ounces of water per day to maintain proper body function. If we add levels of exertion and stress, or extreme hot weather, this number increases. Most people today do not drink enough water on a daily basis, and we generally enter the field in a dehydrated state.

Cardiovascular exercise should be an important part of daily life. If we intend to be active in the outdoors it is not enough to only worry about exercising our circulatory system on the weekends. Simple things like taking the stairs instead of the elevator or parking farther away from the store in the parking lot will help. If you are a daily walker, it will help you to walk with a loaded pack of similar weight to what you would carry into the woods.

If you're confronted with a person suffering from hypovolemic shock, the first step is to stop the bleeding. Then check her airway to make sure it's clear. Elevate her legs 6–12" and keep her warm—and evacuate her promptly.

If the victim has suffered a cervical spine injury, this can disrupt or sever the signals the brain is constantly sending to the heart and blood vessels. As a result, the heart slows and arteries swell. This is *neurogenic* shock. Look for bradycardia (slow pulse), low blood pressure, and neck or back injury. Check for a clear airway, immobilize the spine, and assist with rescue breathing as required. Evacuate the victim as soon as possible. To help prevent this type of shock, if you find signs and symptoms of a spinal injury, immobilize the patient's head by placing a blanket under his neck, then rolling it up to his ears on each side. You should also use a blanket to keep him warm and to restrain his body movement, which could make the injury worse.

If the patient has suffered a heart attack, she may go into *cardiogenic* shock. This makes the heart pump less efficiently, thereby reducing circulation. Signs and symptoms include chest pains; an irregular, weak pulse; anxiety; and cyanosis (bluish color under nails and in lips). There's not much you can do to treat this; the patient should be evacuated for professional medical care as soon as possible. Place the victim in a comfortable state such as seated with hands on knees to relieve chest pressure (tripod position); help her in taking her prescribed medication for the condition. You may also have to help with breathing, which may include rescue breaths.

Anaphylactic shock refers to shock brought on by an extreme allergic reaction. This kind of shock cuts off or constricts airways and dilates arteries. The result is the lungs take in less air, which can lead to mild itching, rash, burning skin, vascular dilation, profound coma, and rapid death. Standard treatment is the administration of epinephrine and the management of the airway.

Anyone who suffers from a chronic allergy probably carries an EpiPen with her; ask where it is, and if she can't tell you, search her pack for it.

If an infection has spread throughout your body, it will probably damage the circulatory system to such an extent that blood circulation will drop. This can send you into *septic* shock. Signs and symptoms include warm skin, tachycardia (rapid pulse), and low blood pressure. The patient suffering from this should be evacuated quickly. While waiting, keep him warm and elevate his feet. This is a good reason to keep close track of any infections and treat them from the beginning.

> **BUSHCRAFT TIP**
>
> Shock can complicate an already delicate situation. If the injury is serious and the patient has lost a lot of blood, anticipate shock. Finish treating other injuries and then assume the patient will go into shock and treat for it.

FOUR STEPS FOR TREATING SHOCK
Here are four things to do for shock:

1. Check the victim's airway and remove any blockages.
2. Perform rescue breathing by giving two normal breaths via mouth to mouth roughly two seconds apart. Aid as needed until the patient's breathing is normal, twelve to twenty breaths per minute.
3. Keep the patient warm by removing any wet clothing and wrapping an emergency blanket, sleeping bags, and hot packs around the patient as needed. In wet conditions erect a shelter to protect the patient, and build a fire if necessary.
4. Keep the person talking. If she passes out, just keep talking to give her something to hold on to, which may aid in her forcing herself back awake.

RECOGNIZING AND TREATING INTERNAL BLEEDING

Unlike external bleeding, which you can see happening, internal bleeding can be easy to overlook—meaning an injured person can potentially lose a lot of blood and go into shock before anyone recognizes the danger.

While internal bleeding can be the result of a number of different problems, such as stomach ulcers, a ruptured ovarian cyst, or an aneurysm (weakened blood vessel), in the wilderness it is more likely to be caused by trauma, such as an ATV accident or a bad fall. Think of dropping a heavy weight on your foot. It might not break the skin but it certainly leaves a bruise! Any type of blunt force like that can create internal bleeding. A fracture can cause damage to the surrounding blood vessels as well, so even if the fracture is closed (doesn't break the skin), internal bleeding may be an issue.

If a person is taking certain types of medications, such as those that thin the blood (warfarin, heparin, even aspirin), or has a medical condition that interferes with blood clotting (hemophilia, liver damage) internal bleeding is more likely and harder to control.

Bruising, swelling, pain, weakness, and dizziness are potential signs of internal bleeding, especially if they occur after an injury or accident. Tenderness, rigidity, and swelling in the abdomen are particularly troubling signs. So too is vomiting or coughing up blood. Over the longer term, black or bloody stools are also a sign of internal bleeding.

If you suspect a person is bleeding internally, check ABCs and repeat them every five minutes. If the person is responsive, raise the legs 8–12" to prevent blood from pooling in the legs and feet, then treat for shock (see "Four Steps for Treating Shock" in this chapter). If the person is unresponsive, place him in the recovery position (see Chapter 3) and treat for shock. Rotate the person to the other side (in the recovery position) every two hours until definitive medical care is available (this will help prevent blood from pooling in one location). In any case when you suspect internal bleeding, arrange for immediate evacuation.

PRACTICAL SCENARIO

While snowshoeing, you find a woman lying across a well-traveled trail with her dog on a leash next to her. As you approach, you don't see any blood on the snow. Her dog leaps about to greet you in a friendly way. Her face looks pale and her eyes are closed. Her respirations are easy, but rapid. You ask her if she's okay as you grasp her wrist to take her pulse.

She responds that something is wrong and that her left side hurts. You mentally note her pulse is strong and fast. You ask her what happened to determine her MOI. She says that she slipped off the ice on the hill just above you and hit her left side hard and that it hurts to breathe. You ask if she was knocked out at all. She replies no and that she doesn't hurt anywhere else. What now?

ANSWER

Introduce yourself and explain that you are trained in first aid and ask if you can further assess her to get a better idea of what's wrong. She welcomes your help. You ask her name, where she's from, the date, and she answers all without issue, which means her mental state is sound. You then ask if you can check her injuries, and she again consents.

You put some freezer bags on your hands to serve as BSI since your snow mittens inhibit movement and feeling. You assess her head, neck, shoulder, and chest and all appear normal with no DCAP-BTLS (see Chapter 3). Both sides of her chest move equally when breathing, so you pull up her turtleneck and unfasten the button of her snow pants to check her abdomen. The upper abdomen looks normal, but as you palpate you discover she's very tender in the left upper quadrant and the muscles are tight in this area, almost rigid. At this point, she begins to vomit in the snow. The vomit has no display of blood and appears to be her last meal.

You stop and think: patient is alert and oriented but her pulse and breathing is fast, though not labored. Her radial pulse is strong.

> Her chest is fine, but her left upper abdomen is tender where she hit when she fell. You recheck the pulse again, counting it this time as 130 beats per minute and it seems weaker than before. Something must be going on internally, such as bleeding, which is making her exhibit signs of early shock.
>
> The best thing for her is immediate evacuation. So you call 911 and treat the patient for shock by keeping her airway open, keeping her talking, and maintaining her core body temperature until help arrives.

SUSPECTED HEART ATTACK

Consider serious disease when a person complains of shortness of breath and weakness, has cold and clammy skin, appears cyanotic (bluish), and has a crushing, tight, or squeezing pain in the chest that may radiate into the neck, jaw, throat, back, arms, and shoulders.

In women, these signs can be more subtle. Often they do not feel the same chest pressure as men do and are more likely to have shortness of breath, nausea and vomiting, and/or jaw or back pain.

Using the SAMPLE history discussed in Chapter 3, find out if the victim has a history of heart disease or heart attack.

> **BUSHCRAFT TIP**
>
> After an angina attack, the person may look and feel normal, but after a heart attack the victim will look sick and be in obvious pain.

An individual who has angina (chest pain that is not a heart attack) will often carry medication to help relieve the symptoms. If this is the case, help her to a comfortable position and assist her in taking her medication. If the medication does not relieve the symptoms, suspect a heart attack.

If you do suspect heart attack, help the person to a comfortable position, sitting or lying, and give one aspirin (if available) or a tea of willow bark to help prevent blood clotting, which can make the heart attack worse. Give water but nothing else to eat or drink. The victim should be carried out immediately.

TIPS AND TRICKS

- Liquid Benadryl ingested moments after an allergic reaction may ease the onset of anaphylaxis.
- Massive blood loss is a major contributor to common injuries that bring on symptoms of shock. Understanding this can be vital to your well-being in the field. Yarrow is a very common plant found in every season that can be used for deep cuts.
- Any plant containing tannins will help stop bleeding, and can be used as a vulnerary (a plant used for healing wounds).
- Don't forget that trees are great medicinals. Many species like oak, walnut, and poplar are high in tannins.

Chapter 8

BREATHING ISSUES

"Regulate the breathing, and thereby control the mind."
—B.K.S. Iyengar

A number of different types of injuries and illnesses can cause breathing difficulties, from the common cold to pneumonia to chest trauma.

TREATING RESPIRATORY ILLNESSES

If you or one of your companions catch a cold, there aren't many treatments other than staying warm and drinking a lot of fluids. Take a decongestant if you have one.

But some respiratory illnesses—such as flu, bronchitis, and pneumonia—are more dangerous. Flu (influenza) is a contagious viral disease that can cause severe illness, even death. It is more dangerous in children and the elderly than in otherwise healthy adults. Although the symptoms of the flu and the common cold can be similar—cough, sore throat—you can tell that you have the flu because it comes on suddenly whereas cold symptoms develop over time. With the flu, one day you're fine and the next you're not.

Be aware when treating someone with the flu that it is highly contagious and airborne (so it's harder to protect yourself from it). You are likely to contract it yourself. Signs and symptoms include a fever, body ache, cough, sore throat, chills, headache, vomiting, and diarrhea. Anti-inflammatory pain relievers such as Advil may help. Mild exercise can also help relieve some of the symptoms. If flu symptoms are serious, arrange for immediate evacuation.

If a cold isn't treated, it can develop into bronchitis, an infection of the lower airways. This isn't too serious (and a good preventative measure is not to smoke, since smoking damages your lungs, making you more susceptible), but it can develop into pneumonia.

Someone with bronchitis will be wracked by a persistent cough and spit up green or yellow sputum that sometimes shows traces of blood. He'll be feverish, lethargic, and congested. As with other respiratory illnesses, rest and plenty of fluids are the best treatment. If the ill person does develop shortness of breath and/or signs of pneumonia, arrange for immediate evacuation.

Pneumonia is an infection of the lungs. There are two kinds: viral and bacterial. Viral pneumonia is generally mild and people recover without any problems. People who contract bacterial pneumonias, however, generally become very ill and need antibiotics to recover.

Pneumonia symptoms (either type) include high fever; productive cough; chest pain, which worsens with deep breathing and coughing; and shortness of breath. One side of the chest may not fully expand during respiration. Like the common cold, pneumonia is irritatingly hard to treat outside of rest, keeping warm, and antibacterial drugs. If the patient doesn't seem to be improving within seventy-two hours, or if the symptoms are severe, you should seek immediate evacuation to emergency care. If you suspect that the victim has bacterial pneumonia prepare for immediate evacuation.

Recently there's been a lot of concern, especially in the southern United States, about the Zika virus. This is transmitted by mosquitoes, and although it shows flu-like symptoms (fever, rash, difficulty breathing, vomiting, chills, sweating, red eyes), it is much more serious. The biggest concern is that it can cause birth defects to children carried by pregnant women infected with the disease.

Currently there is no known treatment for Zika, so if you suspect someone of having it, concentrate on those symptoms you can relieve. Make sure the patient is getting plenty of rest and fluids and use acetaminophen for pain relief. Don't use ibuprofen or aspirin, and evacuate the patient as soon as possible.

TREATING A CHOKING PERSON

If you suspect someone is choking (for example, they are eating or drinking and suddenly start coughing and seem to be having trouble breathing), use the Heimlich maneuver to clear the airway. This involves standing behind the victim, placing your fist just below the sternum in the center of the body, and giving a series of quick abdominal thrusts, using your other arm to hold him in place. This forces air through the airway and can remove any obstacle. Do a quick sweep of his mouth to make sure everything has been removed.

If someone has a partial airway obstruction but can still talk, you should perform the Heimlich maneuver, just as you would if he were fully obstructed.

If a child has an airway obstruction, open the airway by placing your thumb on the tongue and first two fingers under the jaw, pinch together, and lift. If the object is visible, try removing it by sweeping it out with a finger. If you cannot see the object, place the child on her back on a firm surface and provide five abdominal thrusts with the palm of one hand above the navel, but well below the sternum (chest bone). These thrusts will increase abdominal pressure and hopefully move the obstruction into view where you can sweep it out. Only attempt to remove an object you can actually see; otherwise, you may push it farther into the airway. Provide two rescue breaths and repeat this process until help arrives or the obstruction is cleared.

In the case of an infant, rest the baby face-down on your forearm, supporting the jaw and face with your hand. Keep the head lower than the rest of the body. Deliver five back blows between the shoulder blades with the palm of your hand. Place your free hand on the back of the infant's head, sandwich his body, and turn him over. Now take two fingers and give five chest compressions (or upper abdominal thrusts on a larger infant). If you can now see the foreign body, remove it. Repeat the cycle as many times as needed to remove the object.

If after removal of the obstruction the individual—whether infant, child, or adult—remains unconscious, perform CPR if necessary.

RECOGNIZING AND TREATING CHEST INJURIES

Chest injuries are more common than you might think. They are also extremely serious and require evacuation as soon as possible. They can involve damage to the heart and the lungs, two of the most important organs in our bodies. A chest injury can disrupt the victim's breathing, making it too fast, too slow, or irregular. If the heart itself has been injured, it may start bleeding into the pericardial sac (the sac that surrounds the heart). This compresses the heart and may cause it to stop altogether.

OPEN AND CLOSED INJURIES

An open chest wound is one in which the chest cavity is open. Closed injuries are internal. Both kinds of injuries require immediate treatment and probably evacuation.

Sometimes chest trauma results in a sucking chest wound or flail chest, which requires special treatment (see Chapter 4). Signs and symptoms to look for in chest injuries include pain at the site of injury, pain at the injury site made worse with breathing, shortness of breath, coughing or vomiting up blood, failure of one or both sides of chest to expand normally when inhaling, rapid and weak pulse, low blood pressure, and cyanosis of the lips and fingernails (they turn blue).

PRACTICAL SCENARIO

You're assessing a middle-aged woman with chest injuries and difficulty breathing. She hit a tree with her chest while tubing down a snow hill. She has cyanosis around her lips, and her respirations are forty-four breaths per minute, shallow and labored. During the trauma assessment, you ask to unzip her jacket and lift her shirt so you can look for paradoxical motion, which is when the chest moves inward during inhalation (instead of the normal outward motion) and moves outward during exhalation (instead of the normal inward motion). Are there any bruises or deformities? You assure her you are trained in first aid and will keep a blanket over her to keep her warm. The patient refuses to allow you visual inspection. You ask if you can get a woman off the slopes to help aid and she refuses.

ANSWER

The major issues are weather, risk management, and transportation related. Even though the injured woman has an elevated level of respiration and is in obvious distress, if she refuses your help, you cannot provide much more than emotional support until the time comes that she loses consciousness. There will be occasions when an injured or ill person is argumentative and downright combative.

In this case, the cold weather is working against you by sapping body heat away from the injured woman, making her injured body work even harder to maintain homeostasis. Risk management is a concern, because you don't want to leave an injured person unless you have to. Leaving her to get help could encourage her to try and move herself, thereby possibly worsening her injuries. Lastly, making a plan to get her to help is important; so long as she refuses your help, you may have to aid her in moving to get to her preferred help.

SELF-AID

Now, let's say *you* fall out of a tree stand. The strap (which you're supposed to wear!) breaks your fall but does so by constricting around your chest since it slid up violently from your belt line during the fall. Due to the pressure on the snap and your inability to breathe well, you cut the strap with your pocket knife and fall 12' to the ground, which again takes your breath away. You immediately begin to examine your chest as you struggle to catch your breath, and you feel the bottom few ribs sort of floating in place. You find it hard to breathe normal breaths and you're sore. What do you do?

First, try to remain calm. Take a piece of cloth or your hunting pack, dump its contents, and roll it into a ball to place it over your deformed ribs, which may be symptoms of a flail chest. Tape or hold this ball in place as you continue to relax and try to regain a normal breathing pattern. You put the old survivalin' acronym to use—STOP: sit, think, observe, plan. Sit and rest, think about your injuries and assess their severity, observe how you can treat your injuries, and create an actionable plan of treatment and evacuation. Once you do this and treat yourself as best as can be managed, decide if you will be able to attempt self-rescue by walking out. If not, hopefully you know that within a couple of hours after dark, someone will come looking for you if you have taken the time to plan properly. In that case, set up camp, stay warm, and remain calm.

Lung Injuries

Injuries to the lungs will impede normal breathing. If you broke a couple of ribs and one of them penetrated your lung, even though to an outside observer it might seem that there was nothing wrong, inside you the air will slowly drain from your lung until it collapses. Such a condition is called pneumothorax, or "air in the chest."

On the other hand, if there is bleeding into your chest (hemothorax), this can put pressure on the lung and cause it to fail. A symptom of this is that the victim's breath rate increases. The injured party can probably walk out on his own, albeit at a much slower pace than normal.

An injury to the lung may affect more than just the lung. After all, the air is pressing against all sorts of other organs, including the heart. Pressure on the heart, called tension pneumothorax, prevents blood getting to the heart in sufficient amounts. If the victim's neck veins are distended and his trachea is twisted and pushed to the side, he may have this condition. Tap his chest; the injured side probably sounds hyper-resonant.

If this is the case, start plans to evacuate, since the patient will need professional medical care.

TREATING ASTHMA

Asthma is widely spread in the United States; a 2009 study found that 25 million people, or 8 percent of the population, suffer from it. It can include coughing, wheezing, or shortness of breath. Asthma is usually controlled by medication, which is often administered by an inhaler.

Asthma attacks can be mild, severe, or, in extreme cases, life-threatening. Look for shortness of breath and difficulty expelling air from the lungs.

To treat asthma position the victim in a manner that promotes easy breathing (for instance, sitting upright, hands pressed against the knees—this is called the tripod position). Help with any medications, and give the person clear fluids. If, after two hours, the patient is still have trouble breathing, it's time to evacuate.

TREATING HYPERVENTILATION AND SHORTNESS OF BREATH

If someone gets stressed out they can start to breathe far more rapidly than normal (the average person takes between twelve and twenty breaths a minute). If they continue to do this they'll start to feel dizzy and experience a tingling in their extremities. All of this will probably stress them out more, compounding the problem. Since these are also symptoms of heart attack, affected individuals may believe they are having a heart attack. See Chapter 7 for more information about suspected heart attack.

> **BUSHCRAFT TIP**
>
> Respiratory alkalosis, a severe condition, occurs when carbon dioxide levels in the body drop too low, primarily due to hyperventilation. Signs and symptoms include dizziness, bloating, feeling lightheaded, numbness and/or muscle spasms in the hands and feet, discomfort in the chest area, confusion, dry mouth, tingling in the arms, heart palpitations, and feeling short of breath. Treatment requires an increase of carbon dioxide absorption. Having the patient exhale in a paper (not plastic) bag and inhale the carbon-dioxide rich air will aid in reducing symptoms. Providing psychological support will alleviate anxiety.

The best way to treat cases of hyperventilation is to begin by reassuring and calming the victim. If she's stressed out about something in particular, see if you can remove it or remove her from its vicinity. Tell her to take deep, slow breaths. Count them out for her. If she is still hyperventilating, there may be an underlying cause, and you'll have to probe deeper to find out what it is.

TIPS AND TRICKS

- When you use an occlusive dressing to seal a chest wound, note the material used, whether three or four sides were taped down, and any changes observed afterward such as vitals, breath sounds, skin color, and the injured person's level of anxiety.
- To treat hyperventilation, breathe through only one nostril, which lessens the amount of oxygen you're taking into your lungs. For the second approach to be useful, the mouth and the other nostril need to be covered.

- Mullein is a plant with direct affinity for the lungs. You can use this plant for many simple breathing issues that are non-injury-related. Make an infusion (tea) from the leaves of this plant and drink about 8 ounces three times daily until you are breathing better. You can also use this as a vaporizer of sorts by covering the head with a towel and inhaling the steam (at a safe distance).

— Chapter 9 —

NEUROLOGICAL ISSUES

"Take care of your body. It's the only place you have to live in."

—Jim Rohn

While neurological issues tend to be serious, that does not mean you are helpless should one occur in the wilderness without medical help nearby. There are often steps you can take to minimize damage until help can be reached.

IDENTIFYING STROKE

Strokes are more common than we'd like them to be, and they can be quite serious. If someone in your wilderness party suffers a stroke, that person should be taken out of the wild as soon as possible. Sometimes called a cerebrovascular accident (CVA), a stroke interrupts the blood flow to the brain. This, in turn, will often cause slurred speech and loss of function in the limbs.

When they have no blood flow, brain cells die. Even though this process may take a couple of hours, the damage has been done. Occasionally a little blood gets through but it's not enough for the cells to work normally.

There are a few types of strokes, but we will address the most common here.

When there's bleeding in the brain, the victim suffers a *hemorrhagic* stroke. People who suffer from prolonged cases of elevated blood pressure are at most risk for this type of stroke.

If a blood vessel is blocked (for instance, by a blood clot), blood to one part of the brain is cut off. This is called an *ischemic* stroke. Those suffering from high cholesterol or atherosclerosis are at the highest risk for this stroke.

Sometimes when a clot has blocked a vessel, it breaks free quickly. This creates a *transient ischemic attack* (TIA), also called a mini-stroke. It takes about twenty-four hours for normal functions to be restored. TIAs may come as a series of attacks. Any TIA is your body warning you of a forthcoming crisis.

Signs of a stroke:

- One side of the face droops and looks immobile. The victim can't move that side of the face well.
- Arm drifting: if the affected individual holds both arms out with palms up, one arm will drift down.
- Slurred speech: the affected individual has trouble forming normal speech or can't repeat a sentence when asked.

Any person suffering a stroke needs to be evacuated as soon as possible. Place the victim on a backboard with the paralyzed side down. Put a blanket under his head and elevate the head to 6". Describe exactly what happened to the EMS people who are carrying him out.

PRACTICAL SCENARIO

During an outdoor class, one of your instructors suddenly develops a slur in his speech and exhibits a droop to one side of his face and numbness in his hand. He suddenly falls over and as you reach him, he opens his eyes and begins to stand. He walks toward another instructor but in a sideways motion, nearly walking in a circle. What do you do?

ANSWER

As you reach him, you calm him and perform a quick stroke scale: you ask him to smile showing his teeth, which he is unable to do on one side. You then ask him to hold his arms in front of him with palms up. Both arms move, albeit one slower than the other and the slower arm drifts off to the side. Lastly, you ask him to say, "The sky is blue in Cincinnati," which he is not able to do without badly slurring his speech.

He does not pass the Cincinnati stroke scale, so you take vitals and signal to another instructor that immediate evacuation to medical care is needed. A stroke is an emergency, so you should spend as little time as possible where you are in case conditions worsen. Because the affected person is alert and able to walk with assistance, you walk him side by side to meet the ambulance in a nearby parking lot to transfer care.

HELPING SOMEONE WITH SEIZURES

If you are traveling with someone who has a seizure disorder, make sure you understand what his seizures look like (an absence seizure may resemble someone lost in thought whereas a generalized tonic-clonic seizure results in complete loss of body control, convulsions, and unconsciousness). Ask him what to do in the event a seizure occurs.

Most seizures are brief, so if you happen to arrive on the scene of a seizure, it will usually be after the seizure has taken place and the individual is recovering. If the victim is in a dangerous area when a seizure begins, move him as quickly as possible to a safe area. Encourage the victim to sit comfortably and recover. When he's fully responsive, you can begin to discuss what happened. Symptoms of a seizure include repetitive movements of the limbs and inability to respond when spoken to. Seizures that go on for more than three minutes or seizures in pregnant women require immediate medical attention.

> **BUSHCRAFT TIP**
>
> High altitudes, particularly cold atmospheres, can cause seizures even in people who do not have a known seizure disorder and can exacerbate seizures in those who do. Stress, fatigue, and other illnesses or injuries can make a person with seizure disorder more likely to experience a seizure.

If someone is suffering a seizure, start as you would with any injury. Check the airway for blockage. If the seizure has stopped, there's a good chance the victim is breathing heavily and that his heart rate has increased. If these don't start to come back down after a few minutes, something besides the seizure may be going on.

Once the seizure has passed and the affected individual is recovering, perform a physical exam, LOR (level of responsiveness), SAMPLE history, and assess for weakness or loss of sensation in body parts. Keep the patient warm and follow the same procedures you would if he were in shock. Evacuate immediately if the cause of the seizure is unknown or uncertain, the seizure accompanies illness or injury, recovery is delayed, or status epilepticus occurs (that is, seizures continue without recovery between them).

WHAT TO DO ABOUT FAINTING

Fainting is what happens when the nervous system has a sudden reaction that briefly reduces blood supply to the brain. Because of this the brain temporarily stops functioning and the patient faints. People can faint from fear, surprise, bad news, or any strong emotion. Fainting can also be caused by physical conditions such as heart problems.

Fainting is similar to shock, and you should treat it the same way you would treat someone undergoing shock. Once the individual has regained consciousness, recheck vitals and monitor over the next several hours to see if the condition worsens. If vitals remain stable, nothing more needs be done; if, however, vitals decline, look to evacuate.

CARING FOR HEADACHES AND MIGRAINES

Headaches—which we all get at some point—aren't usually taken very seriously; you can relieve them with over-the-counter medicine or by lying down in a dark room for a while. In the wild, the latter option isn't available to you most of the time. There can be many different causes, including altitude, snow glare, or just the exhaustion of your body engaging in vigorous exercise. In some situations, of course, a headache is a sign of something more serious. In any case, a persistent headache should ring alarm bells for you.

Begin by checking for a head injury. Look into the subject's eyes and see if one pupil is dilated more than the other. Feel his forehead. Is it warm? Is he balancing okay?

If the subject is vomiting and hasn't been able to sleep or eat properly, and if this is an ongoing condition, prepare to evacuate the patient. As long as it remains mainly a headache, he can probably walk out under his own power.

Migraines can cause more disability than a typical headache because of their severity and the fact that they often cause nausea and vomiting. These are recurring headaches with pain that is usually focused on one side of the head. They often include light sensitivity, so the sufferer will be more comfortable away from bright sunlight. People susceptible to migraines occasionally report an "aura" (changes in their vision, such as seeing spots) when one is coming on. Individuals with a previous diagnosis of migraine will usually have medication to treat the symptoms; help the person take it. If migraine medication is not available, over-the-counter pain relievers and natural remedies (see Chapter 16) may help.

SELF-AID

Headaches can be brought on because of muscle strain in the neck and shoulders, which can happen when you are exerting yourself in unusual ways. Make sure to take breaks when you're doing unaccustomed labor, and stretch your shoulders and neck regularly. Also, an improperly fitted or too-heavy backpack can bring on headaches through muscle strain. Make sure your backpack fits well and is not overly heavy.

Plants such as willow bark make a pain-relieving tea you can consume to help with mild headaches. A cooling fomentation on the forehead made from a tea (cold infusion) of mint or sumac berries will work to help ease mild headaches as well.

TREATING INJURIES TO THE HEAD AND SKULL

There are two main types of head injuries that involve the brain and the bones of the skull: concussion and skull fracture.

CONCUSSION

A concussion is a brain injury that occurs when a blow to the head moves or shakes the brain, interrupting brain function (often just for a few moments). Back-and-forth movements, like those that happen if you're tackled from behind (such as when playing football) or rear-ended by another car, are especially damaging to the brain. In the wilderness, concussions are often the result of an

ATV accident or a fall. Even a mild blow, such as bumping your head on a tree limb, can cause a concussion.

Any injury that can cause a concussion may also cause an injury to the spine, so check for spinal injury during your assessment. If the pupils fail to respond to a flashlight shined in them, or are unequal, or there is a loss of feeling in the body, or vital signs deteriorate, the person may have a spinal injury.

Although the injured person may "shake it off" and feel okay afterward, do not leave him unattended or let him walk around. The brain may be bruised or bleeding, which can result in confusion, coma, or death.

It's okay to let the injured person sleep, but wake him every two to three hours to check LOR. A headache that gets worse can be a sign of swelling in the brain, causing pressure in the skull.

Treat a concussion as you would shock—protect the airway, keep the person warm, and evacuate immediately.

SKULL FRACTURES

Skull fractures can occur with any head injury, such as from a fall, an ATV or other motor vehicle accident, or from being struck by a falling tree limb or other blow. Like other bone fractures, skull fractures may be open (the bone breaks through the skin) or closed (the bone does not break through the skin).

Check the skull for bone edges, bone fragments, or a depression near the site of the injury. These are all signs that a fracture has occurred. If fluid drips from the nose or ear, it may be cerebrospinal fluid (CSF), indicating a skull fracture or other injury near the spine. To check if a fluid is CSF, take a light-colored cloth and dip a corner into the fluid. If it dries with a yellow halo around the edge, it is CSF; the same yellow halo will occur even if the CSF is mixed with blood.

Cover any open injury with a sterile dressing. Use a doughnut-style dressing to protect the fracture. Evacuate immediately.

TIPS AND TRICKS

- If a person is having a seizure near a cliff or waterway, she should be moved and secured in some way if possible.
- Seizures can result from sudden high fevers in children. Although such seizures are usually well tolerated by children, transportation to medical care is necessary to rule out serious conditions.
- Some people who have had a stroke may be unable to communicate in any way, but they can often hear everything going on around them. Be aware and choose words carefully.

— Chapter 10 —

ABDOMINAL ISSUES

"Those who think they have not time for bodily exercise will sooner or later have to find time for illness."

—Edward Stanley

Organs such as the liver, kidneys, and intestines are often vulnerable to injury both on their own and sometimes from other parts of the body. A broken rib, for instance, can rupture the spleen. If the liver or spleen is badly lacerated, it will bleed heavily, filling internal body cavities and possibly sending the patient into shock. Someone with an injured spleen will probably feel pain in the left shoulder.

If the patient complains of lower back pain, and her urine shows traces of blood, this may be a sign that one or both of her kidneys have been damaged. If the hollow organs such as the stomach or intestines rupture, the patient will suffer intense pain, inflammation, and bloating caused by digestive juices and toxins being released into the body. Such an event can cause infection throughout the lower body cavity. People with serious internal injury will often try to protect the area by holding the stomach/

lying in a fetal position. The abdominal muscles will become very rigid and the injured person cannot relax them (guarding). Blood may also appear in the stool; dark, tar-like blood means bleeding in the stomach or intestines while bright red blood probably just means hemorrhoids.

> **BUSHCRAFT TIP**
>
> Before you begin any vigorous activity, especially one in which a fall is possible (skiing, for example), it's a good idea to empty your bladder. If your bladder's full when you fall, it could rupture and detach from the urethra (the tube through which urine exits the body).

A pelvis fracture can also injure the bladder and the bowels. Sharp bone ends could puncture one or the other.

TREATING OPEN AND CLOSED ABDOMINAL INJURIES

Open abdominal injuries mean there is a puncture or protruding bowel or fat. Closed injuries do not have tears penetrating the abdomen. If the patient has no obvious injuries in the area, take a look at the skin color. Don't confine your examination to the front; also look at the sides and back. Pooling blood, if present, will look like a large bruise on one side of the body. Distension, which in this case is the accumulation of gas or fluid in the abdominal cavity, causes the abdomen to expand beyond its normal girth, similar to pushing your stomach out acting like you're pregnant. Pooling blood, distension, and rigidity are all telltale signs of an internal abdominal injury.

Open injuries require additional protective measures. When something has penetrated the body around the abdomen, do *not* remove it. It's possible that object has sealed a leak in an organ. If you remove it, the organ (especially if it's the liver or spleen) could start to hemorrhage, sending the patient into shock.

Hard as it is, even though something is sticking out of your patient's abdomen, resist the urge to pull it out; instead, pad the area and find a way to hold the padding in place. If you're only moving the injured person a short distance, this will work. If it's going to take a long time, you may have to pull out the object to avoid the risk of infection. You need to watch very carefully for bleeding.

If you're dealing with fat or bowel material that's sticking out through an opening in the skin, you can either try to press the material back into the cavity and then dress it and put a bandage in place to secure it, or you can cover the area with a moist cloth to keep the wound from drying out. Don't push anything into the wound (least of all your finger) and keep the area as undisturbed as possible. Keep the wound moist during transport. Don't push the material in if it's torn, since that could cause it to leak into the abdominal cavity, causing more damage.

> **BUSHCRAFT TIP**
>
> The abdomen is a tricky area, one best left to medical professionals. If the patient complains of abdominal pain, evacuate her as quickly as possible. Don't poke and pry on your own.

If you are not certain of the severity of the injury, watch the injured person over several hours. The pain may become so great the injured party wants to evacuate, or other issues, such as deteriorating vital signs, may occur, which will indicate it is time to arrange evacuation. Alternatively, the injury may not be serious, and as long as the injured person's condition remains stable, evacuation does not need to be rushed.

If the victim has had an internal injury, there may be bleeding and even an infection. Calmly interrogate the patient to find where he's feeling pain and discomfort. Are there external signs such as vomiting? Check the patient for dehydration, particularly in the case of vomiting and/or diarrhea. Feel his abdomen to see if it seems rigid. Is there swelling anywhere?

If yes, evacuate the injured person as soon as possible, because more serious internal injuries that cannot be treated in the field will soon manifest. Treat for shock and evacuate.

In the case of a serious injury, do not give food. The slow sipping of fluid is okay (no alcohol, milk products, or caffeine drinks), and you can give antacids, which will aid in soothing the stomach. For additional comfort, you can use a warmed canteen of water as a heat pad for the area. Be prepared for vomiting, and help the injured person find a position of comfort. Often this will be lying on his side with knees bent. Do not give solid foods or laxatives.

PRACTICAL SCENARIO

You're hiking with your child on a common trail near your home when she suddenly trips and falls onto a broken stump. It lacerates her stomach, and as you roll her over you find that she has intestine protruding through a hole in her abdomen with some blood and a lot of trail debris. She's crying and trying to hold her stomach, so she's alert. You attempt to calm her and fail, but she allows you to treat her. Now what?

ANSWER

You begin by rinsing the debris off her with your water bottle, then carefully lifting her shirt to gain better access to the injury. The hole is small, but with the cool water, cool breeze, and open wound, she's already complaining of being cold. Once rinsed for a second time, the injury isn't bleeding much, so you apply a dampened bandanna to the wound to keep it covered and moist. Because it's not below freezing, there's no reason to attempt to push the protruding intestine back through the abdominal cavity. You apply a second damp bandanna to the wound followed by a used, but clean enough, sandwich bag. You hold it in place because you have no tape and instruct your daughter to hold steady pressure on the wound as you carefully lift her in a cradle carry to get her back to the house where you can call 911.

TREATING NAUSEA AND VOMITING

If a patient is vomiting or is nauseated, this could be a symptom of a larger problem. The first thing is to get the patient to the point she can keep down fluids; otherwise she may become dehydrated. Give her a chance to rest and let her eat small amounts of carbohydrates. She should not have meat or milk for twenty-four hours; if at the end of that time she's feeling better, you can start her on meat, but in small amounts.

These symptoms are associated with many illnesses or injuries, ranging from head injuries all the way to stress. If the patient shows no other symptoms and appears to recover from the nausea, you can continue your hike, but keep a close eye on her.

> **SELF-AID**
> If you suspect you are vomiting or have stomach cramps because of contaminated food or water, charcoal from the fire may be a quick help. Mix charcoal with water in a slurry and consume about 8 ounces. You can eat the charcoal alone, but the slurry is a bit easier to consume quickly. If this makes you vomit do not be concerned, as the charcoal will absorb some of the toxins even if you cannot keep it down at the time.

EASING DIARRHEA AND CONSTIPATION

We're sure that at some point in your life you've had the unpleasant experience of diarrhea. There are many different causes, including food poisoning and various diseases. The big danger to the patient is dehydration, since each bowel movement is releasing a lot of fluid as well as stools. Concentrate on getting the patient safe drinking water. If the patient's urine turns dark yellow, increase the amount of fluids you're giving him. Gradually put him on a carb-heavy diet, avoiding milk and coffee (since caffeine acts as a laxative).

The other side of this is constipation, which can be very painful. Try changing the patient's diet, but stay away from alcohol, bananas, cheese, and other foods that tend to help bind stools tighter together.

HEMORRHOIDS

While blood in the stool can seem like a scary sign, a small amount of bright red blood is likely from hemorrhoids (swollen veins in the rectum) and not from a more serious illness or disease.

Hemorrhoids often develop after constipation, especially if one strains to push out the stool. Make sure the affected person drinks enough water and eats enough fiber, as this can help clear up hemorrhoids.

Sometimes the bowel itself protrudes from the anus (prolapsed bowel), causing discomfort. If this happens, have the affected person get on his knees and elbows with the buttocks higher than the head and apply gentle but steady pressure to the protruding bowel tissue until it slips back inside. Have the person remain in this position (or lie on his side) for thirty to sixty minutes to help make sure the problem doesn't recur.

Dark blood in the stool or black stools are more serious signs and could mean anything from a tumor to an infection, so a consultation with a medical professional is indicated. If abdominal cramping, vomiting, or changes in the vital signs occur along with the dark blood or black stools, seek immediate evacuation as it is possible the affected person could go into shock from blood loss.

HERNIAS

A hernia is typically caused when part of the intestines (or another organ) push through a weak spot in a muscle (often the abdominal wall), creating a bulge. For anatomical reasons, men are more likely to get hernias than women. The most common place for hernias to occur is around the groin/upper thigh, although they can also occur throughout the abdomen. Most hernias do not require urgent treatment. If you or someone in your group is experiencing a hernia and it is causing discomfort, the protruding intestines can often be coaxed back into place if the affected person relaxes and presses them in.

If a hernia becomes strangulated—that is, the protruding intestine or organ is cut off from its blood supply—it requires immediate surgery. A strangulated hernia cannot be pressed back into place, has a firm bulge, and causes increasing amounts of pain. Vomiting may accompany the pain, and the pain may spread throughout the abdomen. There is no effective treatment for this in the wilderness, so evacuate immediately.

TIPS AND TRICKS

- Abdominal injuries are sometimes associated with fractures or traumatic brain injuries. So a thorough physical exam is necessary.
- Keep people with abdominal injuries warm and in the greatest position of comfort. Straightening legs and a lot of movement will increase their pain.
- Open abdominal wounds radiate interior heat quickly, so hypothermic treatment may be required in cold or wet conditions.

— Chapter 11 —

URINARY AND REPRODUCTIVE SYSTEM ISSUES

"It is health that is real wealth and not pieces of gold and silver."

—Mahatma Gandhi

Urinary tract and reproductive system problems can crop up out in the wilderness. These are likely to be illnesses rather than injuries, although injuries to these areas of the body can occur. If that's the case, refer to Chapter 10: Abdominal Issues, for more information on general treatment approaches.

TREATING PAINFUL URINATION

Pain during urination is often caused by some type of infection of the urinary tract. These issues can be eased by drinking plenty of liquids including acidic fluids and juices (such as orange juice or cranberry juice). Avoid sexual intercourse while dealing with any urinary infection.

For urinary tract infections caused by bacteria, antibacterial teas may help. Yarrow and plantain are good choices for this condition. Goldenseal will help stop bacteria from sticking to the bladder walls, helping you avoid infections as well.

Urinary tract infections can turn into kidney infections, potentially damaging the kidneys or causing a life-threatening infection, so medical treatment should be sought if the infection does not clear up quickly.

BUSHCRAFT TIP

It's possible—especially if you're an older man with a history of prostate troubles—that you experience difficulty in urinating. If this happens when you're in the wild, you should avoid drinking fluids until you can either urinate or, more probably, until you can walk out and seek professional medical assistance. Some ways to stimulate urination include:

- Putting your hand in a pot of warm water
- Rubbing the front upper part of your thighs while standing

STAY WELL HYDRATED

Staying well hydrated is essential to urinary system health. The color of your urine shows how hydrated you are. If your urine is clear, you're well hydrated. The less hydrated you become, the darker and more yellow the urine is. (That's why in the morning, after you've been sleeping all night, your urine is generally darker.) If your urine turns brownish, you are severely dehydrated, and it's essential for you to drink some fluids.

PRACTICAL SCENARIO

Your survival class partner has been complaining of a headache, which has been growing in intensity as you continue down the trail. You've been collecting squaw wood for the past hour, and your 55-gallon drum liners are only halfway full, so you have a long way to go before getting back to camp. He suddenly begins vomiting and becomes very lethargic. He says he's been drinking his water but still has three-quarters of a full bottle. He says he's not urinated since he got to class. It's a beautiful day, full sun, and 70 degrees. Now what?

ANSWER

You tell him to drink some more, catch his breath, and relax a few minutes, which he happily does. About ten minutes later he again begins vomiting and can barely walk. Treatment for this patient is rest and rehydration. Once a patient begins to exhibit signs such as these, it's hard to get rehydrated without ample rest, water, and electrolyte intake. Many people operate daily in a decreased level of hydration—urine color should be straw yellow at the least and you should be urinating at least every two hours. Remember, salt and sugar are important too, so eat a light snack while rehydrating to aid in the replenishment of much-needed electrolytes.

COPING WITH KIDNEY STONES

Your party is walking along a path when in front of you a man doubles up, clutching his abdomen. When you reach him to start an examination, he's retching, which soon turns to actual vomiting. As you put your hand on his forehead, you realize he's running a fever. What's going on?

One explanation for these symptoms is the man has a kidney stone. This could be the cause of the sudden pain in his abdomen, as well as the vomiting and fever.

Kidney stones are crystals that form when the body is unable to dilute certain substances sufficiently and they clump together instead of being excreted from the body. Kidney stones can cause a lot of pain. Some stones are too large to pass on their own and require medication or medical procedures (such as shock-wave therapy) to treat.

While making plans for evacuation, increase the fluids the patient is consuming. It's possible that he'll pass the stone, although it's not an experience he'll care to remember. Meanwhile, concentrate on getting him out of the wild as quickly as possible.

> **BUSHCRAFT TIP**
>
> Many field edge plants like gravel root and queen of the meadow have been used for centuries to help break down kidney stones. You can take them as an infusion or simple tea, but they are more effective if the rootstock is used as a decoction.

PAIN IN THE LOWER ABDOMEN

Any sort of severe pain in the lower abdomen is cause for concern, since it may indicate problems with intestines or kidneys and urinary tracts. The safest course is to evacuate the patient. Give fluids as tolerated, treat for possible shock, and evacuate.

MENSTRUAL AND PREGNANCY-RELATED ISSUES

If a woman suffers heavy menstrual bleeding (continuous over twenty-four hours) and she does not have a known medical condition that accounts for it, this may be a sign something significant is wrong. Let the patient rest until the bleeding slows and returns to its normal state. While the patient is resting, give her plenty of fluids. If the bleeding doesn't lessen within twenty-four hours, take steps to evacuate her.

There are several herbal teas that work well for menstrual cramps. Yarrow is one of the best, but raspberry leaves work well too. Black cohosh root is probably one of the most famous, although being a rootstock preparation, it needs to be concocted, not just brewed as a simple tea.

If a woman is pregnant less than twelve weeks, heavy bleeding may signal an ectopic pregnancy (a pregnancy in which the embryo is attached outside the uterus) or a miscarriage. If the pregnancy is more than twelve weeks, the bleeding signals a miscarriage or premature labor. If the woman passes some spongy tissue, she's had a miscarriage. In any case, she should be evacuated as quickly as possible.

> **BUSHCRAFT TIP**
>
> If a man has suffered an injury to his pelvis or spine, one symptom may be that he gets an erection that will not go down. This condition is called priapism and is a sign—if you need one after a spinal injury—that the patient needs to be evacuated.

TIPS AND TRICKS

- When hammock camping, nocturnal leg cramps ("charley horses") are typically due to dehydration. Drink water and maybe have a light snack to replenish salts and sugars for a better night's rest.
- Packets of Jell-O make for an excellent rehydration drink. Add enough to taste in a water bottle and drink. The ingredients aid greatly in replacing lost electrolytes.
- Should you run out of pads during a menstrual cycle, take a folded-over bandanna and place absorbent material (such as moss) inside to serve as a temporary pad.

— Chapter 12 —

ACUTE AND CHRONIC ILLNESSES

"One of the hallmarks of the veteran woodsman is the way he contrives to make himself comfortable in camp."
—WARREN H. MILLER

Many people with chronic illnesses, such as diabetes, can enjoy outdoor adventures with careful management of their situation. The same is true if you happen to come down with an acute illness (a cold, for example). However, sometimes the stress and exertion of being in the wilderness can create a complication with a known illness. In that case, you need to be prepared to take the right steps to deal with the problem.

DIABETES IN THE WILDERNESS

Those who have type 1 diabetes are perfectly capable of going into the wild and enjoying the amazing bounty of nature. They can live healthy, long lives so long as they continue proper treatment. Those with type 1 diabetes may carry an insulin pump to ensure the presence of insulin in their bodies. If you have type 1 diabetes or someone in your group does, be sure to schedule appropriate stops for medication administration and meals.

Type 2 diabetes occurs when the cells become insulin resistant, requiring more insulin to use blood sugar (glucose) as a fuel. Type 2 diabetes can be controlled with a combination of diet and exercise, but with either type of diabetes, the same problems occur when fuel and insulin get out of balance.

> **BUSHCRAFT TIP**
> Diabetics who are involved in physical exercise such as hiking in the wild generally take less medication than those who remain sedentary. In any case, their mealtimes need to be regular.

If you have diabetes, before you leave for your trip into the wild, tell your group leader about your condition. Talk to your doctor about what you should take with you as snacks and food. Be sure to give the group leader the telephone number of your physician in case of an emergency. Bring extra supplies that can be accessed in an emergency, including supplies of insulin.

An emergency diabetic supply may include oral and/or injectable medication and the supplies needed to administer injectable medication (syringes, needles, alcohol wipes). Make sure someone other than the person with diabetes understands when and how to use the emergency kit.

HYPOGLYCEMIA

Hypoglycemia (too little sugar) means that the person with diabetes has run out of fuel. This may happen because the person waited too long before eating or took more of her medicine than was prescribed. Someone who's hypoglycemic will be pale and sweaty. She may feel dizzy, weak, or faint. Her limbs shake, and she's snappish and without much energy. She may drool and complain of numbness in her hands and feet.

Give her some sugar (a very small amount) and watch her closely. If you have a sugar cube, have her put it under her tongue.

HYPERGLYCEMIA

Hyperglycemia occurs when there is not enough insulin to bring sugar (glucose) to the cells, meaning the blood sugar level is raised. This condition is extremely serious, since delayed medical treatment can result in the patient slipping into a diabetic coma.

A hyperglycemic person shows signs of dehydration and dim vision. His skin is red and warm to the touch, and his pulse is weak and fluttery. His breath may be sweet, and he may vomit. He feels intense thirst and needs to urinate often.

The treatment for this condition is insulin. If you don't have any, make immediate preparations for evacuation. While waiting for rescue, have the patient drink as much as possible, since this will reduce the sugar in his blood.

INSULIN SHOCK

If a diabetic misses a meal or accidentally takes too large a dose of insulin, she can experience insulin shock. She'll complain of dizziness and feel sweaty and faint. This is a serious medical emergency, and you should arrange to evacuate the victim immediately.

KETOACIDOSIS

Ketoacidosis is a life-threatening condition that occurs when there is not enough insulin in the body to use blood sugar as a fuel. The body instead uses fat as fuel, which leads to a buildup of ketones, a type of acid, in the body. Someone suffering from ketoacidosis looks much the same as someone with hyperglycemia: he's flushed, his skin is warm and dry, he breathes deeply and fast, and his breath smells fruity. He's extremely thirsty and urinates often. Have him drink a lot of water to wash away the sugar in his blood and prepare him for rapid transport to emergency care as there's no further treatment in a remote location.

ALLERGIES AND HIVES

People with common allergies, such as allergies to ragweed pollen, often avoid the outdoors during prime allergy season to reduce their symptoms. It makes sense for people who have a lot of allergies in the early spring to avoid camping in the early spring. People with plant allergies can also plan to avoid areas that will trigger them. For example, the American Academy of Allergy, Asthma, and Immunology offers an online resource that allows allergy sufferers to see local pollen counts in various parts of the United States and Canada. If you have allergies and know what pollens are most likely to trigger your allergies, you can plan your trip accordingly.

SELF-AID

If you suffer from plant allergies, you can still enjoy the wilderness even if it makes you sneeze. Here are some tips to help you make camping with allergies a bit more enjoyable:

- Prepare your medicine in advance. If you have severe allergies or asthma, bring a first-aid kit with an extra inhaler, epinephrine injectors, and anything else you might need in an emergency. Make sure that your fellow campers know about your condition and tell them who to call and what to do if you experience serious symptoms.
- Keep covered at night. Camping in a good tent can aid in limiting allergens that blow about at night. A tent with a good, tight window screen or hammock with the same technology will enable

you to limit the amount of allergens that come into direct contact with you, at least for your periods of rest.

- Have a cup of tea. Warm teas infused with raw honey, local to the region you're in, will do wonders in alleviating allergy symptoms.

Hives are itchy and annoying and should be taken seriously. They're usually caused by an allergic reaction to something—pollen, plants, food, or insects. Sometimes an infection can produce hives as one of its symptoms. They typically appear as pink blotches on the skin, bumpy and slightly swollen. They normally pass within one day to one week and may become itchy. They can precede anaphylactic shock, so keep an eye on anyone who breaks out in hives. Antihistamines and other topical ointments such as Burleigh Balm are very effective for calming down hives. See Figure 12.1.

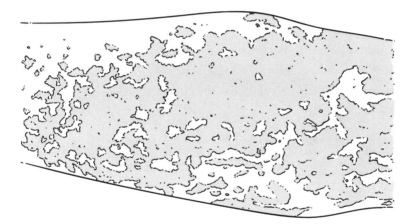

Figure 12.1. Hives on the arm

BUSHCRAFT TIP

Hives, contact dermatitis from plants such as poison ivy and stinging nettle, and heat rash can be treated with antihistamine plants such as jewelweed (they are also anti-inflammatory). Crushing the fresh plant stems and rubbing them on the affected area is good quick treatment.

TREATING ANAPHYLACTIC SHOCK

A severe allergic reaction that occurs immediately after exposure to an allergen such as an insect sting is called anaphylaxis or anaphylactic shock. This life-threatening reaction can close off the airway, making it impossible for the affected person to breathe. Additionally, the shock to the body can cause circulatory collapse.

Signs of anaphylaxis include severe itching or hives; shortness of breath; severe sneezing, coughing, and/or wheezing; swelling of the throat, face, tongue, or mouth or feelings of tightness in these areas; seizures and/or loss of consciousness.

Speed is called for here, since the shock occurs very quickly. Check the patient's airway to make sure it's clear, and do the ABCs. To treat this kind of shock, you need epinephrine. Most people who suffer from known anaphylaxis already have and carry an epinephrine autoinjector with them. These are prescribed medications.

You can use an asthma inhaler or decongestant spray if you don't have access to epinephrine. After the immediate crisis has passed, the patient should take 25–50 mg of Benadryl every three hours for twenty-four hours.

PRACTICAL SCENARIO

A person attending a bushcraft rendezvous begins experiencing shortness of breath and appears to be swelling up and turning red after tasting a plant during a group plant walk. You ask if she is allergic to anything and she replies, "No." Her throat begins to close and she starts to panic as hives begin to appear. Now what?

ANSWER

You happen to have a nasal decongestant spray, so you offer it to her. This seems to help, but not stop, the symptoms. Another person in your group has a first-aid kit containing liquid antihistamine, which you also offer to the affected person. She drinks probably more of it than she should, but it begins to ease her panic and arrest current symptoms. You continue to monitor her airway, breathing, and circulation while instructing her to get into a position of comfort.

Another bystander has gone to get the camp medic, but it will be at least ten minutes before he arrives at the medic station. As you continue to monitor the patient, after five minutes, symptoms appear to have slowed in their progression, but they are still progressing. The person's face and throat are continuing to slowly swell. Without an epinephrine injection, she may not be able to maintain an open airway much longer. Hopefully the medic en route will have some, so you consider having the team move the person, using a stretched blanket and four bystanders in your group, to meet the medic in order to speed the treatment process.

COLD AND FLU

Some tips to remember should you be caught in the field with cold or flu symptoms:

- **Drink plenty of fluids.** Keep a water bottle in hand and make sure no one else drinks from it. Water is the best thing to drink, but watered-down fruit juice can be good, too, as can a cup of tea. If you're unable to keep much water down because of a stomach bug, you'll want to drink something with electrolytes.
- **Have a book or two.** When you're sick at camp you're likely to miss out on activities your friends may be doing, so have a book or two available to occupy your mind between naps. Ample rest is needed for a speedy recovery.
- **Eat, even when you don't want to.** Having some food in your stomach will strengthen your body and boost your immune system, so eat unless you're fighting a stomach bug that rejects everything you attempt to put in it. In those cases, electrolyte-rich drinks are helpful.
- **Let common sense prevail.** If you need rest, rest; if you need a break, take it—don't push yourself beyond your limits while

ill, otherwise you could increase the illness or possibly injure yourself and then have an unnecessary trauma to contend with.

PREGNANCY

Many pregnant women enjoy the great outdoors late into their pregnancies. However, some precautions should be taken. Overheating is dangerous in the first trimester and is suspected of causing abnormal developments in the fetus. Be sure to dress appropriately for where you're hiking.

Exercise is your friend. If you've been exercising regularly during your pregnancy, it's less likely you'll experience any problems in the wild. After the sixteenth week, though, doctors discourage any activity that could result in an injury to the fetus. Falls are more common later in pregnancy because a woman's center of gravity changes and the pregnancy may make movement more awkward. Take special care to avoid falls.

See Chapter 11 for further information on what to do in the case of suspected miscarriage.

BUSHCRAFT TIP You can drink water treated with iodine for several weeks during your pregnancy, but don't do so during the first few weeks; long-term use of wilderness water sources will require alternative methods of disinfection and purification such as boiling.

TIPS AND TRICKS

- You can return the taste to boiled water by shaking it briskly or sloshing it back and forth between two containers to add new oxygen into the water. This will eliminate the flat taste.
- Glucose liquid or a few hard candies are a great addition to anyone's first-aid kit since they will help diabetics and those

of us who get cranky without a little sugar after a hard day's trek.

- Use a powder of white wood ash to help prevent chafing and breakouts of heat rash before a day of hiking.
- When undressing at night, to avoid contact with the oils from poison ivy and other plants (which are surely on your pant legs as well as your boots or hiking shoes), you should remove boots first using gloves if available to unlace them, and then remove pants so that the cuffs do not contact the ankles. Remove socks last. Reverse this order when dressing in the morning if you are wearing the same clothes.

— Chapter 13 —

ENVIRONMENTAL HAZARDS

"People need to be cautious because anything built by man can be destroyed by Mother Nature."

—RUSSEL HONORÉ

Even a well-prepared lover of the outdoors can occasionally get sidelined by an environmental injury—that is, a problem related to weather or the hazards of the local environment. As always, prevention is the best medicine but we've got you covered for those times when it isn't enough.

HYPOTHERMIA, FROSTBITE, AND SUBMERSION INCIDENTS

Some of the most common environmental injuries are related to cold weather. Ideally, you and your group should have the perfect clothing for your stay in the great outdoors, but sometimes the weather changes unexpectedly, or your two-hour hike, for which you're completely prepared, turns into an eight-hour ordeal involving a black bear and an unexpected dive into a lake.

HYPOTHERMIA

When your core body temperature falls below 95°F you are suffering from hypothermia. Untreated, it can lead to severe injury or death. If your temperature is 90–95°F, you are mildly hypothermic, but you should still address the problem immediately. If your core body temperature falls below 90°F you are severely hypothermic.

The first thing to do is to get into warmer temperatures, either by finding a shelter or building a fire. The environment should be dry rather than wet. Eat a carb-heavy diet and stay covered in dry, warm clothing.

Severely hypothermic people are extremely sensitive to touch. If you're administering to one avoid sudden movements of his body. Watch his breathing carefully; you may have to perform rescue breathing.

If the patient's clothing is wet, remove it carefully. Place him on a blanket on top of at least 4" of compressed material so as to insulate him from the ground and wrap him in blankets or spare clothes. Heat metal canteen bottles and put them around his neck and groin, as well as under his arms. Create a vapor barrier from a drum liner or trash bag and wrap him in this. The barrier will trap heat in his body. Evacuate the patient as soon as possible.

SELF-AID

The first step in self-aid is always prevention, but if you start to become cold, shiver, etc., you can check your current state by attempting to touch your pinky finger to your thumb. If you can still do this then you have gross motor dexterity and now is the time to act. Fire is your friend in these conditions. Building a fire and using the reflectivity of a space blanket will help warm you up. Do not sit directly on the cold ground. It takes 4" of compressed insulative material to combat conduction, so take care of that as well. These activities—building a fire, creating an insulating pad for the

> ground—will also increase metabolic heat, which in itself will help as a quick treatment. Make sure you remove and change any wet clothing if possible and also pay attention to a simple acronym (COLDER) when operating in cold environments.
>
> **C** = Clean: Clothing clogged with dirt cannot breathe properly and will trap heat and moisture causing sweat, which can make you feel colder from convection.
> **O** = Avoid overheating: This causes you to sweat, making you colder from convection more quickly.
> **L** = Dress loose and in layers: This helps you adjust clothing easily to release excess heat or trap needed body heat between layers of clothing.
> **D** = Keep clothing dry: This goes back to sweating, but also you need to be attentive to where you sit or kneel.
> **E** = Evaluate your clothing: Review what you're wearing and make adjustments accordingly.
> **R** = Repair: Mend clothing if needed. Clothing with large holes, tears, etc., cannot perform as designed.

FROSTBITE

Frostbite happens when you're exposed to severe cold. When your skin temperature drops below 59°F, your body dilates the blood vessels to pump warm blood to the skin in surges. This is called cold-induced vasodilation (CIVD). If you grew up in a cold-weather climate, your body has likely developed a stronger CIVD response than other people have, and you may be less susceptible to frostbite.

When skin temperature drops to 37–50°F, your body will start drawing blood away from your skin in order to protect the vital organs of the body. When this happens, your skin temperature, particularly in extremities like fingers and toes, can drop as rapidly as 1°F per minute.

Assessing the Severity of Frostbite

There's a tendency, especially among inexperienced outdoors people, to think that numb equals frostbite. The reality is better than that. If your skin temperature falls to 50°F, you'll lose sensation (in other words, become numb). But you're not frostbitten yet. To find out if you're in the early stages of frostbite, use your thumbnail to push down on the area affected. If the skin dents and stays that way, you're heading for frostbite. If you can't dent the skin at all, the freeze has penetrated deeper than the surface layer of skin.

For sufferers from early frostbite, rewarm your hands gently. If you can't dent the skin at all, you'll need medical treatment. The most important thing is to get somewhere warm.

Walking on frozen feet is painful and likely to cause significant damage. For this reason evacuation of the injured person should not rely on him walking if at all possible.

Frostbite Enhancers

Mere cold temperatures sometimes aren't the only factors in creating frostbite. There are several other possible elements. You or someone in your group is more likely to experience frostbite if various contributing factors exist. These include wind chill (the speed and strength of the wind makes it colder); drinking alcohol (something you should never do when hiking in cold weather); smoking (again, not recommended, since it makes blood vessels constrict); hypothermia; exhaustion; imperfectly fitting boots; and wet skin, since any wetness is going to cool things further.

BUSHCRAFT TIP

Remember the old urban legend about a kid who licked a pump handle and froze his tongue to it? Well, there's some truth behind that. If you touch very cold metal, your skin may instantly freeze. That's especially true if you handle a metal fuel container, since petroleum fuels have a lower freezing point. Be smart and always wear gloves in the cold.

Warning Signs of Frostbite

Numbness is your body's warning sign that your skin temperature is getting too low. If you can't get in a shelter or near a fire to warm up, try stamping and wiggling your toes to restore circulation. Put your hands under your armpits or in your pockets. But it can be difficult to rewarm your body once circulation begins to withdraw. Remember the lessons we taught here and in other Bushcraft books about starting a fire under difficult conditions? This is where that training pays off. If you can get them, also keep portable hand warmers in your pack where they're easily accessible.

To treat frostbite, whether in its early or advanced stages:

- Put the affected part, whether hand or foot, in water heated to 104–108°F, which will feel hot but tolerable to the skin. If you cannot tolerate the water, then your patient also cannot, and it will more likely slow-cook the frozen limb rather than aid in recovery.
- If you're the caregiver in this situation, ask the victim to try to move the affected area.
- Warm the hand or foot with heated water for up to thirty minutes or until the skin changes color to red and can be moved and bent.
- When you're finished warming fingers or toes in water, put dressings on them that separate each digit.

Rewarming aims to restore circulation before the tissues are damaged. Tissues need oxygen; without it they can't do their job and they die. So circulation is essential if the patient is going to keep healthy tissues in hands and feet. Properly immersing in water and providing external support by keeping the patient warm, comfortable, and calm is all you can do to ensure circulation returns quickly.

BUSHCRAFT TIP

You may be wondering why we don't recommend a fire as the first step in treating frostbite. The answer is that even though a fire is a good idea, it can't heat the air fast enough to combat tissue damage. Warm water is a more effective immediate solution.

SUBMERSION INCIDENTS

It sometimes happens that a hiker falls through ice and is submerged in cold water for a time. Not only is he cold from the surrounding air, but he is also wet. Combined, these conditions can bring on hypothermia very quickly. Get the person into a warm shelter as quickly as possible and remove his wet clothing. Dry him thoroughly and wrap him in warm dry blankets while setting out his wet clothing to dry. If he has a change of clothing, so much the better. If no fresh clothing is available, a blanket alone is better than wet clothing. Insulative wrap or an emergency blanket are good choices for wrapping the victim, since they'll help his body retain heat. Keep him out of the wind and use a fire with a reflective wall to warm him. Keep a close eye on him to make sure he doesn't develop any other symptoms. Falling through ice can be a very frightening experience. As he recovers, a cup of tea or hot soup is a good idea.

BUSHCRAFT TIP

Chilblains are inflamed areas of skin, usually on the fingers, caused by repeated exposure to the cold, particularly in wet or windy weather. The inflamed skin is red, itchy, and tender. It may blister. Any type of soothing lotion can ease the symptoms. To prevent chilblains, wear gloves. Although chilblains are usually a minor problem, they can sometimes get infected, so keep an eye out for signs of infection (warmth, red streaks, any type of fluid drainage).

PRACTICAL SCENARIO

You and a friend have gone canoeing down the Kentucky River in early March. The weather has started to warm up, with highs in the low 50s, and you both have been looking forward to shaking off your cabin fever. The trip goes off as planned until your buddy decides to get a little overanimated telling a story and lets his paddle go, which results in it floating away quickly. He sees it and scrambles to grab it, tipping the canoe, and you both fall into the cold water. It immediately takes your breath, and you struggle to stay above water; your woolen shirt is becoming heavy and saturated, pulling you down. Your friend was wearing synthetic materials, and he's already made it to shore, so you continue to struggle until your toe touches bottom and you walk up to shore. Your main gear has floated down into an eddy along with your canoe. Your friend is shivering uncontrollably, as are you. Now what?

ANSWER

You instruct him to strip down while you do the same. He's not dressed for the weather, wearing mostly cotton clothes and socks with a thick parka-like jacket. He begins wringing his clothes out. You are wearing wool underclothes, canvas pants, wool socks, and a wool blanket shirt. Since your gear has been lost and you don't have a change of clothing, you wring out your wet clothing and immediately put it back on. Since your clothing is wool, it will retain some of its insulative value even when damp. Your friend, however, is no longer able to manipulate his fingers and cannot unfasten his buttons.

You perform a quick fine-motor skills test and ask him to touch his pinky to his thumb on the same hand, which he's unable to do. Thankfully, you keep a ferrocerium rod in your pocket at all times along with a knife attached to your belt. So, you start a fire within a few minutes. You get your friend next to the fire and begin to heat stones, wrapping them in his wet clothes to aid in drying them out enough for him to put them back on. You feel well enough, so you give him your blanket shirt, which helps him considerably.

His teeth are still chattering, and he's shaking like a leaf, but he's able to speak and barely touch his thumb to his pinky, which is a sign he's improving. As he curls up on the rocky shore, you help him place heated rocks wrapped in his clothing under his armpits and around his core, and he gives a sigh of relief. After about thirty minutes, his clothes are dry enough to put on, and his shivering and chattering has stopped. He's still a little cold but feels much better. You, however, have worked up a sweat trying to care for your patient. Remember, sweat can affect you just as easily when the temperatures are low, so take the time to dry off and cool down before deciding what to do about your canoe and gear.

HYPERTHERMIA, HEAT EXHAUSTION, HEAT STROKE, AND SUNBURN

On the opposite end of the spectrum are the common injuries and illnesses that occur from too much exposure to heat. Prolonged exposure to excessive heat can be just as dangerous as prolonged exposure to excessive cold.

HYPERTHERMIA

The opposite of hypothermia is hyperthermia—the overheating of the body. At 101°F, a person has become hyperthermic. If her temperature stays at 104°F for a length of time, she's in danger of losing her life. When someone is hyperthermic, her skin is hot and dry and she's lost the ability to sweat. Her blood pressure drops and she may show signs of fainting or dizziness.

The first thing is to get out of the sun. If the patient is only mildly hyperthermic, moving her to some shade and loosening her restrictive clothing will help. Keep her hydrated (of course, in the heat, everyone in the party should be focused on hydration). When hyperthermia is extreme and you need to cool her down fast, find a body of water in which to immerse her. Don't expect her to do any swimming on her own. Stand next to her, supporting her. If no body of water is available, put cold metal canteens on her neck and arms.

HEAT EXHAUSTION

Heat exhaustion typically occurs when a person overexerts himself in extreme heat. It can happen anywhere in which the environment is hot and the victim has been engaged in vigorous activity. If someone is suffering from heat exhaustion, you will notice that he seems to be sweating more than usual. As you stop to examine him, he complains of a headache. He appears confused, and his pulse is rapid. He retches violently several times.

The most important symptom of heat exhaustion, and one you must address immediately, is dehydration. Get the patient out of direct sunlight and into a cooler environment. Have him drink as much as possible and if this doesn't result in immediate improvement, give him electrolytes.

HEAT STROKE

If you don't treat heat exhaustion, it will result in a heat stroke, when the victim's core body temperature reaches 106°F. At that temperature cells become damaged, increasing heat production and interfering with circulation, which can hurt internal organs.

- What is referred to as a classic heat stroke (CHS) affects elderly people and those who out of choice or necessity remain in a hot environment. CHS is sometimes called a slow cooker.
- Exertion heat stroke (EHS) happens faster than CHS, sometimes in fifteen minutes. For this reason it's often called the fast cooker, appearing in as little as fifteen minutes; this is typically found in people under physical exertion in extreme heat (hikers, athletes). The symptoms of EHS are similar to those of CHS (heavy sweating), but those suffering from EHS will also have a rapid pulse. If they aren't treated immediately, they will fall into a coma, which can be life-threatening.

Don't be surprised if, when you go to aid the victim of a heat stroke, he refuses to cooperate and even becomes belligerent. This is because with heat stroke, people become disoriented and begin exhibiting an altered mental status, so the first step is to cool him down, either by immersion in cold water or at least getting him away from the heat.

SUNBURN

The most effective way to prevent sunburn is to stay out of direct sun. This seems like common sense, but even when it's a cloudy day, UV rays penetrate the clouds and still do the same harm. When dressing in the summer, wear long-sleeved summer shirts that aid in wicking away moisture while also covering your skin. Also wear wide-brimmed hats, which will protect your head, neck, and face from burning. Cover exposed skin with water-resistant sunscreen—the water resistance is important if you're hiking or working outdoors, since sweat will otherwise sluice off the sunscreen.

Minor sunburn includes redness and relatively minor irritation and can be treated easily enough with skin lotions to soothe them, with aloe-based gels providing a great deal of comfort.

More severe burns that lead to you looking like a cooked lobster will blister and peel. These are actually second-degree burns, and they often cover a large portion of your body. This is why you shiver and get cold so easily when you've got them; you're becoming hypothermic. You may also feel nauseated or have a headache. Sunburns like these will exude moisture, which is the reason your clothing sticks to you after a sunburn. This moisture is your body's natural reaction to burns—it sends plasma to the skin's surface to cool it down. See Chapter 5 for more information on how to treat serious (second- or third-degree) sunburns.

This natural reaction can lead to dehydration over time, so it's important to drink plenty of fluids while sunburned.

Over-the-counter pain medication is helpful as well as aloe-based products or the plant itself applied liberally to the burned area. See Chapter 16 for more information on using plant medicine to treat sunburns.

For other people, these extended periods in the sun not only lead to severe burning, but they cause what we call sun poisoning. Symptoms of sun poisoning include nausea, fever, headache, and dizziness. Move to shelter and drink plenty of fluids; if vital signs deteriorate, arrange for evacuation.

To treat sunburns of any state, follow this same protocol: take a cool (not cold) bath or apply cool compresses to soothe the swelling. Take ibuprofen, aspirin, or acetaminophen to relieve pain.

ALTITUDE SICKNESS

As altitude increases, barometric (atmospheric) pressure decreases. This means that oxygen molecules are spread out more. In other words, there's less oxygen at the top of a mountain than at the bottom. If you're not used to high altitudes, you may start to show signs of altitude sickness. This is particularly true when someone who lives at a low elevation ascends rapidly to a high elevation. Her body does not have time to acclimatize to the new conditions and her body can react in dangerous ways.

If you don't give yourself time to rest and acclimate along the way, even a comparatively low elevation of 6,500' can bring on mountain sickness. If you've ever driven from a low altitude up a mountain (for instance, driving Mount Rainier National Park in Washington State) you know that going too fast creates a headache. You're short of breath, and you may feel lightheaded. This last is a symptom of hypoxia and means you're not getting enough oxygen in your body. Exertion also plays a serious factor in the onset of altitude-induced illnesses.

> **BUSHCRAFT TIP**
>
> Amateur climbers who take inadequate precautions can experience a high-altitude cerebral edema (HACE), a condition that can lead to death. Remaining at a high altitude too long if you're not used to it can also lead to the development of AMS.

PREVENTING ALTITUDE-INDUCED ILLNESSES

To prevent altitude-induced illnesses, there is one medication that can help: Diamox. This helps the body begin producing more red blood cells (the body's main method of dealing with high altitude). This medication must be started at least a week beforehand to achieve its full effectiveness.

The most effective method is to allow your body to acclimate over several days. Climb high, sleep low, is the mantra for this. Take a hike up to 10,000', then sleep at 6,000–8,000' that night. Take a hike up to 11,000' the next day and return lower to sleep again. A few days of this and you will have significantly fewer altitude-related illness issues.

Once on the trail there are a few things you can do to help prevent symptoms from setting in. The first and most important step toward preventing the effects of altitude illness is to drink plenty of water. You will need to urinate more often, and this is the goal since it gives your body more opportunity to expel the excess lactic acid in your system. Slowing your pace will also help since there is less oxygen in the air, and you must reduce your exertion accordingly. Find a pace that works for you.

ACUTE MOUNTAIN SICKNESS

Individuals with acute mountain sickness will display apathy and will have difficulty sleeping. They will complain of headaches and lightheadedness and are likely to lose their appetites. They will be weak and have a poor urine output.

HIGH-ALTITUDE CEREBRAL EDEMA

Individuals with high-altitude cerebral edema will display the same signs and symptoms of AMS, only worse. They'll lose muscle coordination (a very dangerous condition for a mountaineer) and may become unresponsive.

HIGH-ALTITUDE PULMONARY EDEMA

Individuals in the initial stages of a high-altitude pulmonary edema will have a dry, hacking cough and complain of chest pains. Their breathing rate will increase and they will have less energy. As the HAPE progresses, the cough will turn more severe, and they will begin to spit up frothy pink sputum, the product of blood in the lungs. Breathing will become more difficult, and the pulse rate will increase. They will make a gurgling sound when they breathe.

HOW TO TREAT HIGH-ALTITUDE SICKNESS

To treat a person with a high-altitude illness the first step is to recognize the problem. Going higher will make the problem worse, so you should first stop the ascent and then begin to go back down as quickly as possible. If you can administer oxygen, do so. Keep the patient hydrated and give her food (although she may not want to eat). Keep her in the easiest position to breathe; if she becomes unresponsive, she's going into shock and you need to treat for that (see Chapter 7 for information on how to treat for shock).

LIGHTNING INJURY

You may have seen statistics on how unlikely it is that you'll be struck by lightning. That's true, but those who spend a lot of time in the outdoors run a higher risk than stay-at-homes. If you're standing in the middle of an open field during a thunderstorm, you're the most conspicuous object, and you may attract a lightning strike. Water is a conductor of electricity, so it's wise to avoid it in conditions that might produce lightning. The same is true of fence wires. Lightning can jump from one object to another (such as a tree). It can even move through the ground.

The most immediate damage lightning will do to someone is rupture the ear drums. This happens in about half the recorded cases of lightning injuries. Burns, surprisingly, are rarely severe, but your muscles, being subject to a powerful electrical charge, will probably spasm.

To treat someone who has been struck by lightning (or whom you suspect has been struck by lightning) ensure the scene is safe before attempting to give treatment. Move injured individuals to a safer place if necessary. It's possible that several people have been struck by the same bolt. Look after the quiet ones first, since those making noise are apt to have more superficial injuries. Administer rescue breathing to the victim (or victims) until the pulse rate comes down. If no vital signs are detectable, administer CPR. Take into account when doing your examination that the victim's eardrums have possibly ruptured, and he can't hear your questions. You may have to communicate through signs.

Burns and any other injuries should be treated as you would in other circumstances.

FOOD POISONING

Out in the wilderness it can be more difficult to adhere to food safety principles. Sometimes a person will eat something that has been improperly stored or cross-contaminated, and the result can range from a mildly upset stomach to a life-threatening illness.

Carrying unrefrigerated meat for several hours while you travel allows harmful microorganisms in the meat to multiply. While cooking it to well-done can destroy many of those germs, returning the cooked meat to the surface that contains the drippings—and the germs from the raw meat—can then contaminate the cooked meat. This is just one example that most campers, novice and advanced alike, are guilty of. It can and often does lead to illness, but it can all be avoided by implementing the following tips:

- Wash your hands frequently when handling food, especially after handling raw meat. When soap is not available, potable water alone is better than nothing. Consider using wood ash as a disinfectant. It can easily be rinsed off.
- Insulated thermal containers and coolers keep food hot or cold for many hours. Pack coolers so that meat drippings do not contact other food. Keep coolers wrapped with towels or blankets to increase their ability to keep items cold or hot and keep them hidden from direct sunlight.
- Preservative-rich foods such as salt-cured meats, processed lunchmeats, and hot dogs are slow to spoil and retard the growth of harmful microorganisms.
- The best way to transport raw meat for long distances is to start out with it frozen solid. Ground meat will thaw faster and is more perishable than solid pieces and therefore should be the first item cooked. Cook meat thoroughly to the center (medium-well to well-done). Place cooked pieces on clean surfaces. Wash utensils after using on raw and cooked items, and eat the meat while it's still hot.
- Charcoal is your friend—should you become ill after ingesting food, crush some charcoal into a fine powder, add it to water, and consume the mixture. It will aid in arresting microorganisms and bacteria in your digestive system, which will make you feel much better.

EYE INJURIES

Eye injuries are not uncommon in the outdoors. When you're hiking up a trail, you might be watching your footing and not notice the tree limb until it slaps you in the face, injuring your eye. Or, you might be warming yourself by standing close to the fire and a spark finds its way into your eye. When hiking with others, use trail etiquette by holding limbs and other potential sources of injury out of fellow travelers' path. Consider wearing safety glasses or even dust goggles while trekking through thick brush if you don't have sunglasses or do not wear prescription lenses. Protective eyewear, while not always fashionable, certainly beats a stick in the eye. Debris from fires, dust, and trees can all factor into eye injuries as well—little bits of bark or dust from the fire under the eyelid can drive you nearly mad while also scratching the cornea. There are three types of eye injuries common to wilderness travel:

DEBRIS UNDER THE EYELID

When debris is under the eyelid, it scratches the surface of the eye and is very irritating, leading to itching, redness, swelling, and a plethora of tears. To treat, first clean your hands before attempting to flush the eye with clean, potable water that is lukewarm or near body temperature. If something is really stuck under the eyelid, fight the urge to rub it, thereby potentially grinding it into the eye. Instead, ask someone to lift the eyelid to locate it (it may be attached to the eyelid, so if you're treating someone else, look carefully and have the affected person look in all four directions, as it sometimes moves with the eye). Roll a piece of gauze or soft cotton and dampen it, then place it under the person's eyelid and drag it toward you to scrape out the debris. Should that not work, pad the eye and tape it closed, and evacuate the injured person for medical care.

CONJUNCTIVITIS (PINKEYE)

Pinkeye is an inflammation or infection of the transparent membrane (conjunctiva) that lines your eyelid and covers the white part of your eyeball. It can be caused by allergies or a bacterial or viral infection. Pinkeye can be extremely contagious and is spread by contact with eye secretions from someone who is infected. Symptoms include redness, itching, and tearing of the eyes. It can also lead to discharge or crusting around the eyes. Generally it will clear on its own within two weeks.

Allergen-induced pinkeye can be treated with antihistamines such as diphenhydramine (Benadryl) but bacterial infections require antibiotic drops. Avoid getting it by washing your face with potable water, and do not open your eyes underwater while in the field. Unclean water, rich with fecal bacteria, is a leading reason why this ailment is contracted in the wild. It's a good idea to rinse your eyes with eye drops after spending time in a particularly dust-ridden area or taking a swim in a questionable water source.

PENETRATING EYE INJURY

A penetrating eye injury is when the eye itself has been penetrated by being lacerated or impaled by an object. It's a very serious injury requiring immediate evacuation. If lacerated, control the bleeding and heavily pad the injured eye. You may instruct the injured person to close both eyes, which will limit movement of the injured eye, but this also means first-aiders will be responsible for evacuating him since he'll be unable to walk out on his own.

Should the eye be impaled, do not remove the impaled object, and instruct the injured person to resist the urge to remove it. Control the bleeding, pad the object to inhibit movement by rolling gauze pads, socks, T-shirts, or any other cotton material available, and tape it into position. Once the object is secured, consider the object's length. If it's too long to allow for safe evacuation, you may have to shorten the object. Avoid, if at all possible, sawing motions when shortening and, again, only shorten if absolutely necessary. Again, the injured person should close both eyes so the injured eye is not forced to track with the open eye. Evacuate to medical care as quickly and safely as possible.

TREATING DEHYDRATION

You may have a mental picture of sitting by a crystal-blue lake, sipping a cup of water you've just drawn from it as you gaze at the herd of deer drinking a dozen yards away. That's a nice picture, but get rid of it. In fact, fresh water is often contaminated.

Biological pathogens are the main water concerns if you're traveling in the United States and Canada. You can use a water filter to get rid of protozoan cysts (such as *Cryptosporidium parvum* and *Giardia lamblia*) and bacteria (such as *E. coli*, *Salmonella*, *Campylobacter*, and *Shigella*).

Water purifiers go a step further by also combating viruses (such as hepatitis A, rotavirus, and norovirus) by the addition of chemicals such as chlorine or iodine, or UV light. If you're traveling in less-developed areas of the world, consider using a water purifier rather than relying on a water filter alone.

Prefiltering is another important thing to consider. If you're gathering water that is cloudy or silty, UV light purifiers and ceramic-style filters will not work as effectively, and the water may require multiple treatments. Boiling water remains the most low-cost and effective means of making water potable. At elevations under 10,000', bringing water to a rolling boil (boiling about one minute) is all that's required. In elevations above 10,000', add one minute of boil time for every 1,000' of elevation, not to exceed twenty minutes. So at 14,000', you would boil for four to five minutes. Boiling the water and using a UV light or iodine will eliminate all potential contaminants, but this is overkill for much of the United States and Canada; you can generally get by with one or the other without issue unless you're in a chemically contaminated area such as an industrial or agricultural runoff zone.

Straw filters (plastic pipe filters meant for one person to use) provide a lightweight, quick way to get water into your system, but only in small quantities. While this is fine when you're on the move, it's not good for a base camp or when you're camping over multiple days. Also, when it's cold, straw filters can shatter if dropped or freeze up altogether if not properly cared for.

The key to remaining hydrated is to begin your trip fully hydrated. On your way to your destination, you should be drinking water every fifteen minutes or so until you get there. You should have already devised your water plan for the trip beforehand, so if you're going to carry in 2 quarts of water (about 4 pounds) and rely on nature to provide the rest, have the appropriate gear to get water fast (such as a straw) and in large amounts (such as a gravity filter) for when you're in camp.

Multiple containers such as stainless steel bush pots make boiling several servings of water at one time a cinch. But don't wait until you're dehydrated and thirsty to begin boiling; it's already too late and you're likely not going to catch up and rehydrate properly unless you spend a full day in one location boiling water in larger amounts (10 cups at a time). It's not the boiling that's difficult, but the cooling—it takes water longer to cool than it does to bring it to a boil—so consider placing the boiled container in a cooling puddle at the side of your water source. This will help speed the cooling process and aid in getting water into your body faster.

Remember that overhydration is also dangerous as it can lead to hyponatremia. With this condition, the body holds on to too much water. This dilutes the amount of sodium in the blood and causes levels to be low. Symptoms include nausea, headache, confusion, and fatigue. So if you're taking the time to rehydrate, but hit a point at which you begin forcing water into your system and start feeling tired and nauseous, ease off. Limit your fluid intake and rest. Hospitalization may be needed in advanced cases.

TIPS AND TRICKS

- Plants that provide mucilage (slimy texture) such as violets and mullein will aid in soothing a sunburn when applied topically.
- A cup can be placed over an object impaling an eye to serve as a protective covering for the eye and a brace for the impaled object.
- Space blankets with reflective side up can provide good shade from the sun.
- Cotton is not the best wear for cold-weather environments, but to take advantage of evaporative cooling in the summer, there is nothing better than a cotton T-shirt.

— Chapter 14 —

INSECT AND ANIMAL BITES

"In my life outdoors, I've observed that animals of almost any variety will stand in a windy place rather than in a protected, windless area infested with biting insects. They would rather be annoyed by the wind than bitten."

—TIM CAHILL

What's a camping trip without a few chigger bites? While most encounters with insects are more annoyance than injury, sometimes you will need to treat an insect bite (or at least soothe the sting). As unlikely as it may seem, insect stings can be more dangerous to you than animal bites!

PREVENTING INSECT BITES

You may never be able to completely foil the chiggers, but you can take some steps to reduce the likelihood of insect bites and stings. For example, be aware of where you are walking, sitting, standing, and sleeping. You don't want to make your bed over a fire ant colony.

APPROPRIATE CLOTHING

Clothing is your first line of defense against the elements, including insects, and is considered one of the Ten Cs—a cover element. Therefore it is also part of your shelter considerations. Appropriate clothing for wilderness travel will vary slightly with the changing seasons but will always include a base layer and middle layer (which may serve as an outer layer in warmer months) and in cooler months, an outer layer or shell as well.

SELF-AID

Long-sleeved shirts and long pants, even in summer months, will help protect you from insect bites. Tuck pant legs inside boots and then use duct tape for garters. This will help keep ticks from the legs. Mosquito netting can be placed around the head and face and can double as a minnow net for fishing. Many plants have a natural bug repellent factor. These include most with a volatile oil, such as birch. Many plants like yarrow can be rubbed on the skin as a raw plant and will do some good as well. One of the best things is a clay-based mud smeared on any exposed parts of the body.

BATTLING INSECTS

We need to distinguish between insect repellents and insecticides. Repellents are substances we put on our skin. An insecticide can't be put on your skin; it's for use on other materials (clothing, tent walls, etc.).

While the most widely used repellent is DEET, be careful! Using it in too high of concentrations on your skin can bring on an allergic reaction. Be cautious of using it on small children. These days a number of repellents are manufactured specifically for kids. Keep the repellent away from your lips, eyes, and any cuts or scrapes you have.

In the battle against ticks, chiggers, fleas, sand flies, and mosquitoes, the best insecticide to use is permethrin. Never put it on your skin; use it only for clothing, tents, sleeping nets, or shoes. Since it retains its power for weeks and even months, you probably won't have to apply it more than once or twice a season. As well, it won't stain or injure the fabric. Put DEET on your skin and permethrin on your clothes and tent and you're likely to avoid the problem of insects.

IDENTIFYING AND TREATING SPIDER BITES

Spiders may creep a lot of people out, but the vast majority aren't dangerous. Some are venomous, and a very few are dangerous to humans. Most spider bites aren't a cause of concern. A few spiders do have fangs long enough to pierce human skin and venom toxic enough to make humans sick. These include the black widow, tarantula, and brown recluse spiders. It's extremely rare to die from a spider bite in North America but the venom can make you sick enough to warrant professional medical attention.

When you're bitten by a spider, you'll probably feel a sharp prick followed by a red mark where you felt the pain. If the spider is venomous, the bitten person may experience muscle stiffness and cramps in the bitten limb. These may gradually start to affect other areas of the body such as the abdomen and chest as the venom progresses through the body. As time passes, other symptoms manifest themselves:

- Aching and itching
- Fever
- Heavy sweating
- Headache
- Weakness
- Vomiting
- Joint pain
- Rash
- Severe abdominal pain

If someone in your party has suffered a bite and begins to show these symptoms, clean the bite, using soap and clean water. Then put cold packs on the bite; this will help ease the pain. If you don't have over-the-counter medication to address the situation, look for tulip poplars and make a poultice from the leaves. You can also do this with plantain or black walnut leaves. If the bitten person is showing signs of poisoning, check her airway regularly and begin preparations for evacuation. Doctors will administer an antidote to the bite and will almost always do this to children and elderly people. Try to find the body of the spider that administered the bite, although this will probably be difficult. The body will help doctors determine what kind of spider bite they're treating.

THE BLACK WIDOW

The black widow is one of the most widely known of poisonous spiders, although relatively few people have seen them in the wild. They're found throughout the world, but humans are only affected by the bite of the female. Females have a red spot on their abdomens; it's shaped rather like an hourglass. See Figure 14.1.

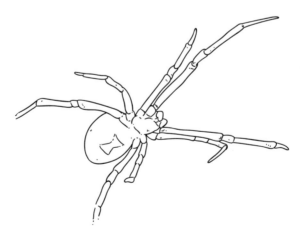

Figure 14.1. Black widow spider

BROWN RECLUSE SPIDER AND HOBO SPIDER

The brown recluse has a uniform body color (ranging from cream to dark brown). Its back has a purplish-shaped marking that looks a bit like a violin. This gives it its popular name: fiddleback. While they are most common in the southern and central regions of the United States, they're also found in northern areas. Similar to the brown recluse is the hobo spider, found in Europe and Asia as well as the United States and Canada. It has no markings, and even though its bite is poisonous, there is a lot of debate in the scientific community about how dangerous it really is. If nothing else, the bite is very painful. See Figure 14.2.

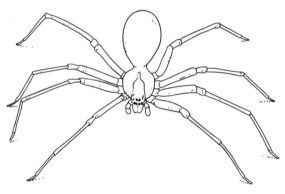

Figure 14.2. Brown recluse spider

TARANTULAS

When we think of big hairy spiders, we're probably thinking of tarantulas. They have distinctively hairy bodies and legs and can range in length from about 4.5" to 11". Though their bite is painful, the venom is weaker than the venom a bee carries in its stinger, so it is unlikely to cause any problems unless you happen to be particularly allergic to them. You are more likely to have a complication because the bite itself hasn't been properly cleaned than because of the venom. See Figure 14.3.

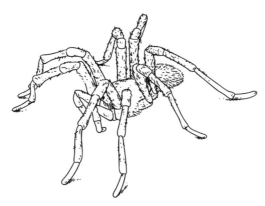

Figure 14.3. Tarantula

IDENTIFYING AND TREATING TICK BITES AND TICK-BORNE ILLNESS

The danger of tick bites is that they're painless. This may sound like an odd thing to say, but the real danger is that if a tick bites you and attaches itself to you, you can carry it for days before you're aware of it. Since ticks are potential disease carriers, this is serious. This is why it's important to do frequent visual inspections when you're out in the wilderness. Be sure to pay special attention to areas prone to tick bites, such as the ankles and neck.

While most ticks are harmless, some carry Lyme disease (LD) and Rocky Mountain spotted fever. A few can cause tick paralysis. The best defense against tick bites is not to let them land on you. Ticks are heaviest in clearings near woodlands—such as trails, paths, and open areas that are frequented by larger animals, so pay special attention when traveling in these areas. Wear clothing suitable for keeping ticks off: long-sleeved shirt, long pants, hat. Consider using a combination of pesticide and insecticide as described in the "Battling Insects" section earlier in this chapter.

If these measures fail, the next step is to remove any ticks before they have time to infect you—thus the importance of the daily skin check. The longer a tick remains attached, the greater the likelihood that you'll develop an infection. Ticks can be difficult to remove once they've attached themselves to your skin. Make sure you've removed the entire tick. Sometimes the body pulls away, but the head remains, which can still cause an infection.

REMOVING A TICK

To remove a tick, use tweezers to grasp the tick as close to the skin surface as possible. Pull it out of the skin using a steady motion and even pressure. If the body detaches, leaving the head buried in the skin, remove the head with a needle or some other sharp instrument, since the head can still cause infection. If you don't have tweezers available, use your fingernails but be sure to protect your hands with gloves (remember the importance of body substance isolation).

Once the tick is removed, wash the bite with soap and water. Use cold packs or a cold canteen to help reduce swelling and to relieve pain. The signs of infection from a tick bite may take a while to appear—as much as a month from the time of the bite. If you develop a severe headache or fever, see your doctor immediately.

> **BUSHCRAFT TIP**
> Ticks have a four-stage life cycle: egg, larva, nymph, and adult. Eggs hatch into larvae, larvae become nymphs, and nymphs grow into adults. After they hatch, ticks require blood to survive at every stage of development.

Lyme disease, one of the fastest-growing infectious diseases in the United States, is a bacterial infection that is passed on to humans by the bite of a tick. It's most commonly carried by the deer tick. The nymph of the deer tick is the most prevalent carrier.

Because it's only the size of the period at the end of this sentence, it is difficult to see. See Figure 14.4.

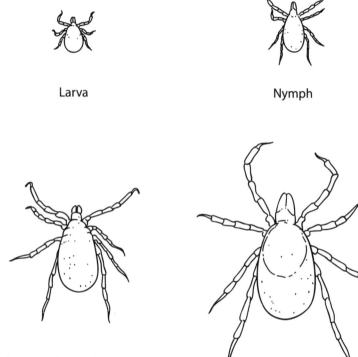

Figure 14.4. Deer tick

LYME DISEASE

Lyme disease–infected ticks are prevalent all over the United States but are more commonly found in the Northeast and Upper Midwest.

Symptoms can take several weeks to develop and people often don't make the connection between the onset of the illness and the tick they removed weeks ago. The early symptoms of Lyme disease are similar to the flu—fever, chills, muscle aches, and nausea.

Joint pain is also common. If not treated, inflammation from the disease can spread to the nervous system and other organs. Sometimes (though rarely) the damage is permanent.

If caught early enough, Lyme disease can be treated with antibiotics and won't cause lasting damage. Treatment is usually effective in stopping the progress of the disease even if it isn't diagnosed immediately, but some people may experience symptoms for months or years after treatment.

ROCKY MOUNTAIN SPOTTED FEVER

Like Lyme disease, Rocky Mountain spotted fever is a bacterial illness that people contract from infected ticks. And like Lyme disease, the symptoms can take a while to present themselves, in this case from about two to fourteen days after the bite. Symptoms include fever, muscle aches, abdominal pain, vomiting, and headache. Sometimes a rash occurs a few days after other symptoms begin.

Ticks infected with the Rocky Mountain spotted fever bacteria can be found throughout North America but are especially common in the southeastern United States.

As with Lyme disease, early treatment (within the first few days of symptoms) with antibiotics usually results in a cure. Because Rocky Mountain spotted fever can be quite serious and is potentially fatal, if you experience any flu-like symptoms after a tick bite, be sure to seek immediate medical attention.

IDENTIFYING AND TREATING INSECT STINGS AND INSECT-BORNE ILLNESS

Although people are more afraid of snakebites than bee stings, they're actually more likely to die of a bee (or hornet or wasp) sting than a snakebite. Some people are so allergic to stinging insect venom that a single sting can be fatal (anaphylaxis, which is discussed in Chapter 12). It's possible to develop an allergy at any time in life even without a previous history, and multiple stings can be fatal even if a person is not allergic to the venom.

People are most commonly stung by honeybees, yellow jackets, wasps, and fire ants, so take care to build camps in areas free of these insects. Become familiar with their habitats. For example, fire ants tend to build their characteristic colony mounds in open areas. Honeybees prefer living near wildflowers and will build their hives in trees nearby. Wasps make hives in trees, shrubs, and on the outside of buildings.

PRACTICAL SCENARIO

You're on the trail in a wooded area with some hiker friends when you feel a sting at your neck. You slap at it but whatever bit you is gone. At first you assume it's just a mosquito bite but the sting gets worse as you continue to walk—way more pain than a mosquito would cause. Now what?

ANSWER

You ask one of your hiking buddies to take a look at the site of the bite. When he does so, he notices a stinger in the bite site. No one has a pair of tweezers along but you have a sail needle in your backpack, and he uses that to scrape out the stinger. You don't have any history of allergies to bee stings. Once it's out, you feel some relief, although the site of the bite is still sore. You clean the bite with soap and clean water, then hold a cold compress against it for about fifteen minutes, and that helps with the pain. Your buddy keeps an eye on you for the next hour to make sure you don't develop an allergic reaction.

People can usually tell when they've been stung by a stinging insect. To treat a sting, first remove the embedded stinger (if there is one), then wash the site of the bite with soap and water. To reduce swelling and pain, apply ice or a cold canteen to the bite for fifteen minutes or so. If the bite itches or causes pain, over-the-counter pain relievers and antihistamines can help provide relief. Keep an eye on the patient for at least one hour after the bite. If he shows signs of a serious allergic reaction, such as hives, redness, swelling all over the body, or difficulty breathing, administer epinephrine immediately if available. In any case, maintain the airway and evacuate immediately.

SNAKES AND SNAKEBITES

Poisonous snakes are the staple of fiction and nightmares. However, of the vast number of snake types in the United States, only two families are poisonous: pit vipers and coral snakes.

Pit vipers, which include copperheads, rattlesnakes, and water moccasins, have a triangular, flat head, wider than the neck; vertical elliptical pupils; and a heat-sensitive "pit" located between the eye and nostril. They can range in size from 1–12', but on average they tend to be 3–4' long.

The coral snake, on the other hand, is small. Its name derives from the colorful bands of bright red, yellow, and black that encircle its body. The red banding is bordered by yellow banding against black. The coloring is similar, but not the same, to the nonvenomous king snake, which has red and black bands. When in doubt, remember the rhyme, "Red on yellow, kill a fellow; red on black, venom lack." Coral snakes are far less likely than pit vipers to bite and unlike pit vipers tend not to strike repeatedly.

A quarter of the time when a venomous snake bites someone, it doesn't inject any venom. The bite is painful, but there's no poison in the system.

SYMPTOMS OF SNAKEBITE

The symptoms of snakebite include pain or burning sensation where the bite occurred. Looking closely, you'll see two puncture wounds where the fangs broke the skin. Within a few minutes the area will start to swell, and the skin will discolor. The area around it will show signs of blistering, and the victim may feel nauseous and start to vomit. If the bite is not treated, this can escalate to bleeding. Eventually the victim will slip into a coma and may die.

TREATING SNAKEBITE

The most important aspect of treating a snake bite is to attempt to get as much of the poison out of the victim's body as possible. Suction the bite with a Sawyer Extractor if you're carrying one (a wise choice for your pack if you're traveling in an area where snakes are prevalent); if not, don't try to use other means of suction. If the symptoms are escalating, you need to get the victim out of the wild and to a medical professional as soon as possible. However, evacuation should be done by moving the victim as little as possible, since activity will help spread the poison throughout the body.

A doctor will treat the bite with antivenin, but this must be administered within four to six hours of the victim being bitten, so time is important here. You can put the bitten arm or leg in a sling to immobilize it and walk the person out.

Monitor a bite victim closely. If no symptoms appear after six or eight hours, he's been fortunate to have been "dry bitten" with no venom in his body. On returning home, he should get a tetanus shot.

There are some definite *don't*s when it comes to treating a snakebite. One of the biggest concerns is the popular myth about sucking the poison from the bite with your mouth. Don't do it. Don't put a tourniquet on the bitten limb, either. It's unlikely to stop the poison from spreading, and it could do further damage. The skin around the bite is in a very delicate condition, so don't treat it with ice packs. And don't let the victim drink alcohol or take aspirin, both of which thin the blood, which will make it easier for the poison to spread throughout the body.

ANIMAL BITES

Most of the time in the wild, you won't get near enough to animals for them to bite you. However, you should know the treatment for animal bites on those rare occasions when it happens. (This treatment applies to domestic animals as well, of course, so the next time your dog or cat nips you, you'll know what to do about it.) Animal teeth will leave tears and punctures in your skin. Although the bite itself may not be dangerous, if it's not treated properly it can become problematic. Clean, dress, and bandage the wound and monitor it carefully for any signs of infection.

RABIES

The biggest danger from the bite of a wild animal is rabies, a serious brain infection. However, you can take some comfort from the fact that North America is at a low risk for rabies, according to the Wilderness Medical Society. According to the Centers for Disease Control, only one to three cases of human rabies are reported each year in the United States. Despite the unlikelihood that you will contract rabies in North America, consider the possibility if you're bitten by a dog, cat, skunk, raccoon, or fox and the attack has been unprovoked. As well, you may be at risk if you're bitten by a bat or a large carnivore. Rabies can also enter your body through open wounds, if a rabid animal licks it.

Any sort of bite in the wild should be treated seriously, and the victim should be evacuated so that she can be given anti-rabies serum as soon as possible.

TREATING ANIMAL BITES

To treat an animal bite victim, wash the bite vigorously with soap and water, use an antiseptic on it, dress and bandage the wound, and seek immediate medical care, noting the animal that gave the injury. If the animal is dead, bring it with you so its brain can be examined for signs of rabies. If it's not dead, try to capture or kill it.

TIPS AND TRICKS

- Many snakes emit a cucumber-like smell when touched or disturbed, so if you smell this odor in an odd location, keep a watchful eye.
- Do not make a habit of reaching for rock ledge handholds while climbing in warm weather as snakes choose these areas often for shade.
- When stepping over logs be sure to look on the opposite side before stepping to ensure a snake is not present.
- Black widows love woodpiles and dead logs, so when harvesting from these locations for resources wear gloves to help avoid any issues.
- An immediate spit poultice of plantain is never a bad idea for any type of bite.

Chapter 15

POISONOUS PLANTS

"Poison is in everything, and no thing is without poison. The dosage makes it either a poison or a remedy."

—PARACELSUS

Though you probably won't suffer any long-lasting effects from a close encounter with poison ivy, the immediate symptoms of pain and itching can make it impossible for you to enjoy your time in the great outdoors. In this chapter, we'll look at plants that are poisonous to touch. Chapter 16 offers precautions so that you don't accidentally eat a poisonous plant.

As with all wilderness injuries, prevention is the best medicine, so learn to identify potentially harmful plants before you engage in outdoor activity, especially in overgrown areas. Wear gloves and long sleeves, do not make contact with your face or eyes with gloved hands, and do not wipe your face on your sleeve. Carry a solvent such as alcohol sanitizer, which will cut the plant oils that induce a contact dermatitis.

Don't forget about what happens at night. When you've tracked through poisonous plants all day long and then reach down to get undressed for the evening, guess what you are doing? Spreading the poisonous plant oils to anything you touch. Here are some things to think about:

- Always remove boots first with your gloves on (if you are highly allergic).
- Wear slip-on boots instead of laces if you can.
- Next remove your pants, not your socks, as removing the socks will rub the cuff of the pants against the skin, again spreading the oils.
- Socks come off last and go on first in the morning.

PLANT-RELATED SKIN CONDITIONS

Many people—about 70 percent of those in the United States—have a sensitivity or allergy to a compound called urushiol present in the resin of certain plants. After touching (or brushing against) plants such as poison ivy, susceptible people develop contact dermatitis, which is an inflammation of the skin that causes redness, itchiness, and blisters. While contact dermatitis is not dangerous, it can be painful and the itching can be extremely uncomfortable. If scratching the itches leads to breaks in the skin, it is possible to get an infection.

The most common cause of contact dermatitis in the United States is just three plants: poison ivy, along with poison oak and poison sumac. You can encounter poison ivy almost everywhere in the United States except Alaska, California, and Hawaii. Poison oak is much less common and is more likely to be found on the coasts (the West Coast more so than the East Coast). Poison sumac is generally found in the southeastern United States.

BUSHCRAFT TIP Though the blisters that form after contact with a poisonous plant are filled with fluid, this fluid does not contain the allergen itself and doesn't cause the allergic reaction to spread. Contact dermatitis itself isn't contagious and you can't spread it to other people. It's the *resin* from the plant that contains the allergen and causes the reaction to spread. Since the resin is sticky, it tends to remain attached to surfaces (including skin and clothing) and can easily spread to other surfaces (and other people) you might touch after exposure, such as clothing, bedding, and even your pet. Wash your skin and any clothing you were wearing and be sure to clean any surface that may have come in contact with the resin.

RECOGNIZING POISONOUS PLANTS

Here's a brief introduction to identifying poisonous plants and treating their poisons.

POISON IVY

You may remember the old saying, "Leaves of three, let it be." That's still excellent advice. Poison ivy plants usually have clusters of three broad leaves shaped like spoons. Once you know what it looks like, it's easy to spot—and you'll spot it everywhere. Poison ivy can be a vine or a shrub; the vine can grow low to the ground or it can climb on fences or trees, so you have to keep an eye out for it constantly. See Figures 15.1, 15.2, and 15.3.

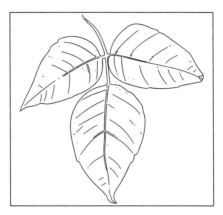

**Figure 15.1.
Poison ivy**

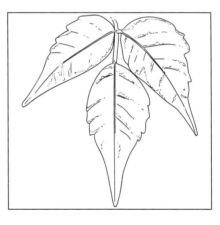

**Figure 15.2.
New leaflets
are shiny and
pointed**

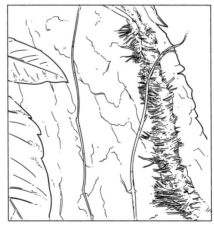

**Figure 15.3.
Reddish rootlets
anchor poison
ivy vines to the
tree's bark**

POISON OAK

Poison oak gets its name because its leaves look like oak leaves—slender leaves with scalloped edges. The leaves grow in odd-numbered groups of three, five, or sometimes seven. In the spring it produces yellow-green flowers that become berries of a similar color in the summer. Like poison ivy, it can grow as a vine or a shrub. See Figures 15.4 and 15.5.

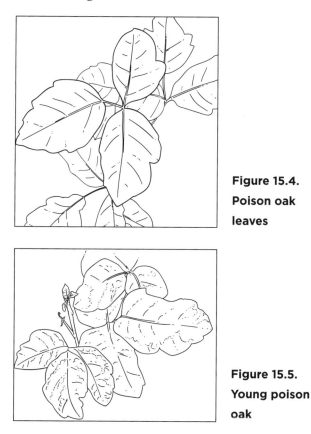

**Figure 15.4.
Poison oak
leaves**

**Figure 15.5.
Young poison
oak**

POISON SUMAC

Poison sumac can be a tree or a shrub, and can grow quite tall—20' or more. Typically the foliage is not very dense. As a small plant, the leaves grow upward but the branches sag down as the plant reaches full height.

Leaves grow in parallel pairs up the stem with a single leaf at the end of each stem. Stems can be red, brown, or gray, depending on the age of the plant. The leaves have an oval shape that comes to a point at the ends. As with any deciduous plant, the leaves change color as the seasons change. See Figures 15.6, 15.7, and 15.8.

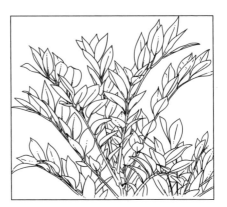

**Figure 15.6.
Poison sumac**

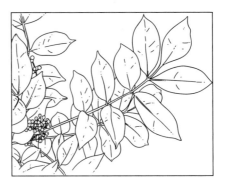

**Figure 15.7.
Poison sumac**

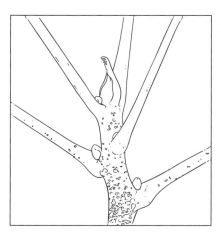

Figure 15.8.

Stem of the

poison sumac

TREATING REACTIONS TO POISON IVY, POISON OAK, AND POISON SUMAC

If you touch any of these plants, their resins will begin to bond to your skin. The process takes about half an hour, so if it's been more than thirty minutes since you made contact with the plant, it will take more than soap and water to remove. So it's important to wash your skin immediately after exposure and to remove and wash any of your clothing that came in contact with the resin as well (being careful not to touch the surface with your bare skin).

If you are not able to immediately remove the resin, use an alcohol-based cleaner or a commercial preparation (Poison Oak-n-Ivy skin cleanser, for example). To treat:

- Wash hands and infected surfaces immediately with soap and plenty of water. Isopropyl alcohol (in hand sanitizers) works great for neutralizing the resin as well.
- Apply calamine lotion if available.
- Burleigh Balm and Fix'n Wax also work to slow spread and itching if applied regularly.
- Jewelweed and plantain also aid in the prevention of spread, redness, itching, and swelling.

SELF-AID

If you're suffering from an itch because you got too close to a pile of poison ivy, any plant or tree with a high concentration of tannins will constrict the pores of your skin and help push the oils to the surface where they can be neutralized more easily or scrubbed off. Oaks, both red and white, have high concentrations of tannins even in the leaves. You can create a cold infusion or a tea that will help as a wash. However, do not use warm liquid on an itch as this will only serve to aggravate the condition.

PRACTICAL SCENARIO

You're out clearing shooting lanes for the upcoming deer season. It's hot out and you're reduced to using a pruning saw since your chainsaw has been giving you fits. You're sweating profusely, but are well hydrated, so you keep about your business. You spot some poison ivy, which you're allergic to, on the tree you're cutting and make every effort to work around it. A limb you cut off falls harmlessly to the ground but brushes your face and arm on its descent. You continue for the next couple of hours until you're finished at which point you notice that your arm is pink and slightly swollen in a small spot and your face has a slight tingle, although not an itch yet. Now what?

ANSWER

You are quick to realize the branch that brushed your face earlier may have had some ivy on it that you didn't see. Under normal conditions, a simple brush may not have affected you, but because the pores of your skin were opened due to the heat and excessive perspiration, they more readily absorbed the oil from the plant.

You go home and wash your face and hands with Dawn dish soap (which helps dilute the oils), then jump into the shower (which opens your pores). You get clean and feel better, but now you have a pronounced itch and swelling on your face with bumps appearing on your arm. You apply some poison ivy cream, which alleviates the itch, and take an antihistamine to boot, but it's too late—you got poison ivy that easily and just have to ride it out.

TIPS AND TRICKS

- Lye soaps are very good on cases of contact dermatitis such as this as they are drying to the skin and will help neutralize the oils through the alkaline content of the soap.
- Be very careful not to burn cut wood that has ivy vines attached as inhalation of the smoke from these oils can be very uncomfortable and even deadly for someone very allergic.
- Some people can develop life-threatening allergies when exposed to poisonous plants even though most people aren't seriously endangered by them. Keep a careful eye on anyone who develops contact dermatitis from a plant and seek immediately medical help if any symptoms of a severe allergic reaction occur (shortness of breath, wheezing, difficulty swallowing). Most allergic reactions occur within twenty-four hours of exposure.

— Chapter 16 —
PLANT MEDICINE FOR THE WOODSMAN

"You know what they call alternative medicine that's been proved to work? Medicine."

—Tim Minchin

Sometimes the easiest and best medicine to find and use in the wilderness is the one growing at your feet. For thousands of years, people have used herbal remedies to deal with injuries and illnesses. With some education, you can learn this lore.

When considering the common ailments of the traveler in the woods, we are not looking to cure or treat serious disease, we are looking to aid our comfort level from common injury and sickness such as a shallow cut, sore throat, or upset stomach. This is where understanding simple plant and tree medicines can come in handy.

To get started in herbalism, you should understand that in an emergency situation, the best herb you can have is the one you have at hand. You must get creative with application and use, and you must be proactive in picking herbs as you see them in your outdoor excursions, before they are actually needed.

BUSHCRAFT TIP

Remember that plants are often a resource that can be used only two or three seasons out of the year, but trees are always a four-season resource. For the majority of common complaints, a tree can be found that is comparable in properties and action to most plants.

Many times plants grow in an environment that may give you a clue to their use. For example many plants that grow in moist areas are mucilaginous or slimy. Plants growing in open fields of full sun are usually dry and act as a drying-up agent. The other thing to keep in your head from the ancients is called the doctrine of signatures. According to this theory, plants may look similar to an organ of direct affinity or resemble a symbol that we are familiar with. For example, the back side of the leaf of the mullein plant greatly resembles the look of the lungs, and this plant is known far and wide to help with breathing and opening the lungs. A plant like goldenrod, which has a jagged and pointed leaf like a knife or spear, is known to be good as a styptic for stopping shallow-wound bleeding.

SELF-AID

In the bush, you are really looking for "simple." This boils down to one ingredient or plant that will address a single symptom or condition. This is a bit counterintuitive from modern herbalism, which often relies on combinations of plants. However, it is much less complicated and allows you to use resources available on the fly. For example, if you break out in a rash and you think it is from poison ivy because you have been seeing it all day in the area you are walking, the simplest approach is just to treat the symptoms. Jewelweed has properties within the plant that are both anti-inflammatory and anti-histamine. This mucilaginous plant grows in wet areas along creeks and often in areas where poison ivy is prevalent, so you can find a patch nearby and simply use the plant stems crushed for topical application. It takes just a few minutes. This simple approach will help relieve at least temporarily the major symptoms of the reaction.

TREATING BY TISSUE STATE

The woodsmen of the eighteenth, nineteenth, and early twentieth centuries could go out into the woods and find the medicinal plants they needed to survive. We've lost much of this knowledge over the years, but the following will give you the essentials needed to treat common ailments with plants typically found throughout the Eastern Woodlands.

By learning to treat by tissue state (as described by herbalist Matthew Wood), you remove a lot of the guesswork involved in selecting treatment options so long as you can positively identify your medicinal plants.

> **BUSHCRAFT TIP**
>
> What are herbs? The botanical definition is a seed-bearing plant that dies back to the ground after blooming and does not have a woody stem. The other definition of herb, which is the one we will use in this chapter, is any plant or part of a plant that is used for medicine. Under this definition, herbs include leaves, flowers, buds, stems, roots, bark, berries, seeds, mushrooms, rhizomes—any plant or part of a plant that can be used for healing.

THE FIVE TISSUE STATES

The five tissue states are:

1. Dry: dry cough, first-degree burns, and abrasions
2. Cold: constipation, fungal infections
3. Wind: changing conditions of hot/cold, cramps
4. Hot: minor burns, fever, bites, blisters
5. Wet: bleeding, diarrhea, wet cough/congestion

Once you understand tissues states, you can select a plant to treat the tissue state, regardless of the specific problem. The herb can treat any of these issues—the processing of that herb is really all that will change.

HERBAL PROPERTIES

Please note that you should not go around tasting plants that you cannot readily identify. When you begin to study plants and learn to identify them, it helps greatly to find a local expert you can work with. If one is not available, all is not lost. You can learn on your own, but you should follow a few simple rules.

Get at least three references that show the plant in detail and have a good description of not only the plant itself but also where and how it grows. Photos of it in different parts of its life cycle will be very helpful. When it comes to trees, be sure to get a book that shows details of the bark, nuts, and fruit as well. Take your books to the field and start exploring.

> **BUSHCRAFT TIP**
>
> One acronym I learned from a man they call Green Dean is ITEM:
>
> - I = Identity: Identify the plant with several references.
> - T = Time: Is the plant growing, blooming, fruiting in the proper time of year?
> - E = Environment: Is the plant growing in the proper environment?
> - M = Method: Use the proper method of harvest and preparation.

Understanding herbal properties will allow you to understand how to apply a medicinal plant to a specific tissue state. For example, different plants have different taste properties that will treat a specific tissue state:

1. Mucilaginous: sticky, slimy—used for lubrication and cooling
2. Bitter: bitter flavor—used for stimulation and heating
3. Astringent: dries out the mouth, creates a pucker reflex—used for drying and restricting
4. Volatile oil: fragrant plants—used for soothing and antisepsis
5. Resin: sticky substance that hardens, such as pine sap and birch tar—used for antisepsis and as an antifungal

PLANTS FOR

DRY CONDITIONS

SWAMP VIOLET (*Viola palustris*)

Taste: Mucilaginous

Areas found: Violets are found all over North America

Description: Blooms from the end of February to the end of April. In the Eastern Woodland variety, the flowers are a deep purple and the leaves are heart shaped, up to about 2" across, with a single leaf on each stem.

Medicinal actions: Aromatic, soothing odor, slimy feeling on the skin

Uses: It can alleviate symptoms of dry tissues, such as a dry sore throat, a dry cough, and sunburn. Aids in regulating the digestive system, such as bloating, gas, and constipation (it is mildly laxative).

See insert, page 1

SASSAFRAS (*Sassafras albidum*)

Taste: Root-beer flavor, spicy, and mucilaginous

Areas found: Throughout the Eastern Woodlands

Description: Sassafras is a very common tree in the Eastern Woodlands, having three different leaves: one with a single lobe, one that resembles a mitten, and another with three lobes. These trees grow erratically and will almost never be straight when mature.

Medicinal actions: Carminative, moistening, lubricating

Uses: Settling an upset stomach, relieving inflamed eyes, relief of menstrual cramps. Root bark is a blood thinner and taken often in the spring can help cool the body over the season. A poultice of this tree's bark is great for deep bruises to help dissipate the blood. Pregnant women should not take sassafras.

See insert, page 1

PLANTAIN (*Plantago major*)

Taste: Moistening, fibrous, bland

Areas found: Throughout most of the United States, in disturbed soil especially

Description: There are two main species in the United States: the long- or narrowleaf plantain (*lanceolata*) and the wide-leaf species (*major*). Both have the same general uses. It grows close to the ground. The most distinguishing characteristics for identification are the large veins on the back of the leaf, and also the spike that rises when the plant goes to seed. With wide-leaf plantain, when you tear the leaf the veins contain a thread-like fiber that will becomes exposed as well.

Medicinal actions: Best used as a drawing poultice

Uses: Treats infection or venoms from under the skin, as with an insect sting, or festered splinter.

See insert, page 1

NETTLES (*Urtica dioica*)

Taste: Bitter

Areas found: Damp draining areas near lowlands in rich soil

Description: Grows in patches generally. It has rough leaves with stinging spines on the stem of the plant.

Medicinal actions: Diuretic, tonic, astringent, anti-allergenic, and anti-inflammatory

Uses: Nettles can be useful in cases of hay fever and allergies, as well as skin problems. If stung by nettles, you can squeeze a little of the leaf on the sting for relief.

See insert, page 1

CATTAIL (*Typha latifolia*)

Taste: Mucilaginous

Areas found: Generally in water edges or very damp drainages

Description: Easily identified by the large brown cob-like flower head at the top of the plant, cattail has many long green narrow leaves layered from the base of the stem.

Medicinal actions: Antiseptic, pain reliever

Uses: The jelly that grows between young leaves can be used to relieve pain and as an antiseptic. The pounded roots can be used as a poultice for burns and sores, the down can be used as a binder or dressing for wounds, and the inner juices used as topical anesthesia and antiseptic.

Other plants that can be used to treat dry conditions:

- Shepherd's purse
- Slippery elm

See insert, page 1

PLANTS FOR COLD CONDITIONS

BONESET (*Eupatorium perfoliatum*)

Taste: Acrid (irritatingly strong)

Areas found: Damp meadows and lowlands

Description: Blooms from July to September. The distinguishing feature of this plant is that the stem appears to grow through a single opposing lance-shaped leaf. Its flowers are white but this is true of many plants; the leaf structure is the best way to identify this plant.

Medicinal actions: Warming, stimulant, laxative when taken in excess

Uses: It can help cold tissue states, such as cold, flu, mild hypothermia, and constipation. If skin tissues show decreased oxygenation (pale, gray, blue, purple tint to skin), it can be used to stimulate the person. There's an old folk term, "bone-break fever," which refers to this plant. It is well known for raising core temperature to help break a fever and fight off infection.

See insert, page 2

DOGWOOD (*Cornus florida* L.)

Taste: Acrid, foul

Areas found: In most areas on edges of the Eastern Woodlands

Description: Flowering dogwood has a white to pinkish flower in the summer and has a dark and heavily segregated bark. It grows very twisted and never straight. Often it will lean toward a clearing or field edge and generally has a low crown. The berries on this tree are red, many times in clusters of four.

Medicinal actions: Warming, stimulant

Uses: Fever with chills.

See insert, page 2

GOLDENROD (*Solidago rugosa*)

Taste: Dry

Areas found: Open fields, roadsides

Description: Long-stemmed plant with lance-shaped leaves. Many species differ slightly, but all have a large cluster of yellow (gold) small flowers.

Medicinal actions: Astringent, antifungal, anti-inflammatory, diuretic

Uses: Goldenrod is used on the skin to heal wounds and is taken internally to reduce bloating.

See insert, page 2

RED CLOVER (*Trifolium pratense*)

Taste: Sweet, cooling

Areas found: Most woodland edges and fields, in disturbed areas

Description: Red clover usually has three leaves, typically shaped like a shamrock, with a red/purple color flower in season.

Medicinal actions: Male/female tonic

Uses: Used for hot flashes/flushes and PMS, as well as lowering cholesterol, improving urine production, and improving circulation of the blood, to help prevent osteoporosis, reduce the possibility of blood clots and arterial plaques, and limiting the development of benign prostate hyperplasia. Red clover is a soothing lymphatic for sore throats and coughs. It is also antispasmodic, making it useful for spasmodic coughs resulting from bronchitis. It is gentle enough to use on children.

See insert, page 3

CHICORY (*Cichorium intybus*)

Taste: Bitter

Areas found: Disturbed soil, especially near roadsides

Description: Chicory is a long-stemmed plant with a pale blue to purple flower that only opens in the daylight.

Medicinal actions: Tonic, laxative, diuretic, sedative

Uses: It can ease digestive problems and improve function, prevent heartburn, reduce arthritis pains, detoxify the liver and gallbladder, prevent bacterial infections, boost the immune system, and reduce the chance of heart disease. It is also a natural sedative, can protect against kidney stones, and can help you lose weight.

See insert, page 3

RIVER BIRCH (*Betula nigra*)

Taste: Acrid

Areas found: Wet areas; it is a water-indicator tree

Description: River birch has a white color bark on the outside, typical of birch but more red underneath and peeling in small chips, not in larger sheets like many birch.

Medicinal actions: Diuretic, antirheumatic, stimulant, astringent, anthelmintic, sweating agent

Uses: An infusion made from the leaves of the birch can be used as a diuretic and cleansing agent to the urinary tract. In addition, it has been used to treat gout, rheumatism, and mild arthritic pain.

Other plants for cold tissue states:

- Shepherd's purse
- Mustard
- Horseradish
- Alfalfa

See insert, page 3

PLANTS FOR
WIND CONDITIONS

MULLEIN (*Verbascum densiflorum*)

Taste: Flowers are sweet, leaves are bitter

Areas found: Throughout North America in areas characterized by gravel, sand, or chalk

Description: It flowers during July and August. The leaves are often described as lamb's ears; they are soft and furry, slightly delicate-feeling, although they are quite strong. A pale green to gray-green color is normal, with a second-year stalk bearing yellow flowers rising from the center rosette to more than 6".

Medicinal actions: Anti-inflammatory, antibacterial, absorbent (when using raw leaves)

Uses: It can be used for wind conditions, such as chest colds, tension in the chest, sudden changes endured in body temperature (such as a submersion incident), chills, and joint pain. It can help treat gas and bloating that comes and goes suddenly as well as nausea and vomiting. The leaves of the mullein make good natural gauze and absorb blood well. It is fantastic as a wound dressing due to its inherent antibacterial properties. Mullein can serve as a sanitary pad and toilet paper.

PRACTICAL SCENARIO

A fifty-eight-year-old man has a head cold that seemed to be getting better. Suddenly the symptoms have gotten worse. He is having unstoppable coughing jags. He can't sleep because of the coughing and feels miserable. What should you do?

ANSWER

Administer mullein with boneset (about equal parts) in a tea, taken as needed to relieve symptoms. After a good night's rest, it is likely that the affected individual will wake up on the path to improvement.

See insert, page 4

BLACK WILLOW (*Salix nigra*)

Taste: Acrid

Areas found: Generally a water-indicator tree and found in moist soil areas and water-holding depressions

Description: This tree often leans. It has deeply furrowed gray bark and plentiful lance-shaped leaves with fine-toothed jagged edges.

Medicinal actions: Analgesic, anti-inflammatory, appetite depressant, astringent

Uses: Willow bark acts a lot like aspirin, so it is used for pain, including headache, muscle pain, and menstrual cramps. Willow bark is also used for fever, the common cold, flu, and weight loss.

See insert, page 4

WHITE WILLOW (*Salix alba*)

Taste: Acrid

Areas found: Generally a water-indicator tree, and found in moist soil areas and water-holding depressions

Description: The white willow is similar in appearance to the black willow except its leaves have a fine white fur-like growth that is predominant on the underside.

Medicinal actions: Antifever, pain reliever, anti-inflammatory

Uses: White willow reduces inflammation and fever, and it is a mild pain reliever. It is useful for gout, back pain, and arthritis.

See insert, page 4

TULIP POPLAR (*Liriodendron tulipifera*)

Taste: Intensely acrid

Areas found: Throughout the Eastern Woodlands

Description: Tulip poplar is a very tall tree, usually the tallest in a canopy line looking from afar. Generally the branches will fall off and die below the canopy level making for a long, straight grayish trunk with obvious eye-shaped scars where branches have dropped. When turned upside down the leaf of this tree looks a bit like a nightshirt—hence the folk name mother-in-law's shirt.

Medicinal actions: Astringent, warming

Uses: The inner bark of the roots is used as a diuretic, tonic, and stimulant. A tea is used to treat gastrointestinal problems, rheumatism, coughs, and fevers. Externally, the tea is used as a wash and a poultice on wounds and boils.

Other plants for wind tissue states:

- Valerian
- Chamomile
- Wild lettuce
- Blessed thistle

See insert, page 4

PLANTS FOR HOT CONDITIONS

CURLY DOCK, A.K.A. YELLOW DOCK
(*Rumex crispus*)

Taste: Sour

Areas found: Edges of woodlands, pastures

Description: This plant is easily distinguished in two seasons: In the summer, the leaves are long and lance-shaped and twist in a curl, giving it the nickname curly dock. The leaves are dark green and fairly rough with a red vein in the center. In the late summer it is one of the first plants to turn almost completely dark brown.

Medicinal actions: Anti-inflammatory, with warming properties that drive fluids to the skin's surface for cooling effects

Uses: It can be used to treat mild hyperthermia, swelling, and inflammation. It can reduce tenderness associated with autoimmune disorders.

See insert, page 5

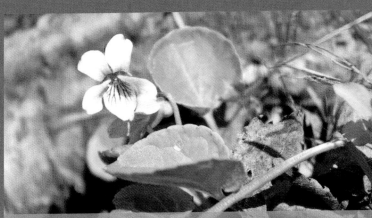

Swamp Violet (*Viola palustris*)
Alleviates symptoms of dry tissues, aids digestion

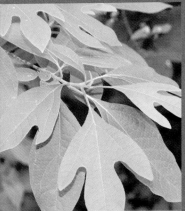

Sassafras (*Sassafras albidum*)
Carminative, moistening, lubricating

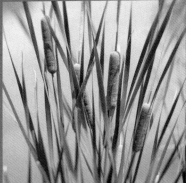

Plantain (*Plantago major*)
Treats infection

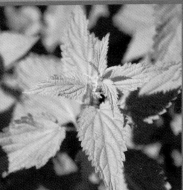

Nettles (*Urtica dioica*)
Diuretic, tonic, astringent, anti-allergenic, anti-inflammatory

Cattail (*Typha latifolia*)
Antiseptic, pain reliever

1

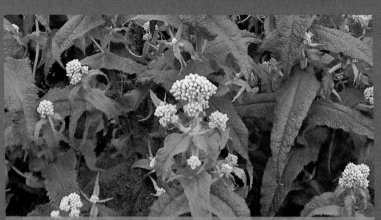

Boneset (*Eupatorium perfoliatum*)
Helps with cold, flu, mild hypothermia, constipation

Dogwood (*Cornus florida* L.)
Warming, stimulant

Goldenrod (*Solidago rugosa*)
Astringent, antifungal, anti-inflammatory, diuretic

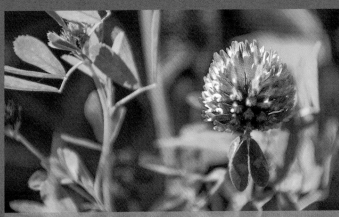

Red Clover (*Trifolium pratense*)
Male and female tonic

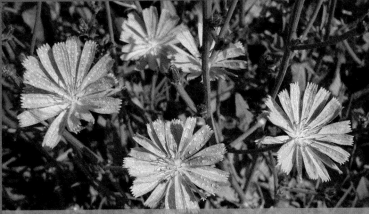

Chicory (*Cichorium intybus*)
Tonic, laxative, diuretic, sedative

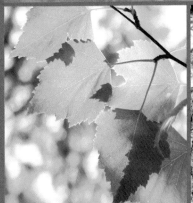

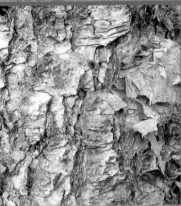

River Birch (*Betula nigra*)
Diuretic, antirheumatic, stimulant, astringent

3

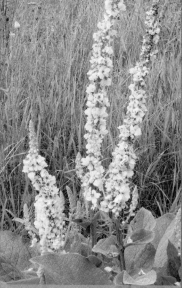

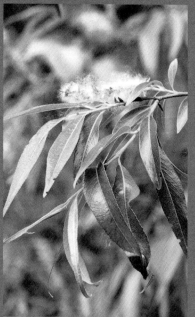

Mullein (*Verbascum densiflorum*)
Anti-inflammatory, antibacterial,
absorbent

Black Willow (*Salix nigra*)
Analgesic, anti-inflammatory, appetite
depressant, astringent

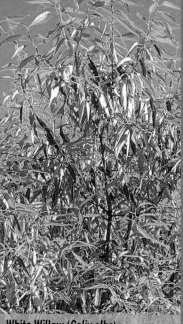

White Willow (*Salix alba*)
Antifever, pain reliever, anti-
inflammatory

Tulip Poplar (*Liriodendron tulipifera*)
Astringent, warming

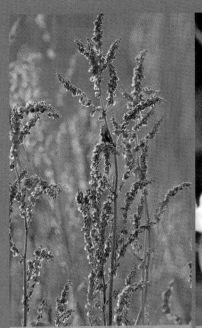

Curly Dock, a.k.a. Yellow Dock (*Rumex crispus*)
Anti-inflammatory, cooling effects

Honeysuckle (*Lonicera*)
Antibacterial, anti-inflammatory, antispasmodic, diuretic

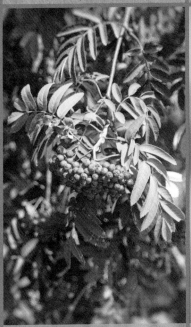

Black Cherry (*Prunus serotina*)
Astringent

Wood Sorrel (*Oxalis stricta*)
Cooling, tonic, anti-inflammatory

5

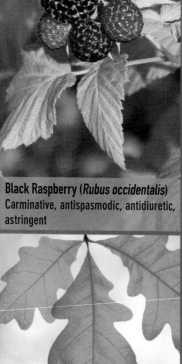

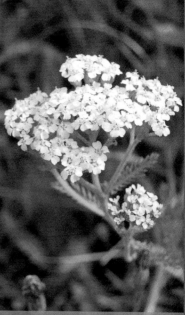

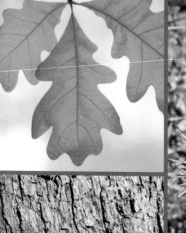

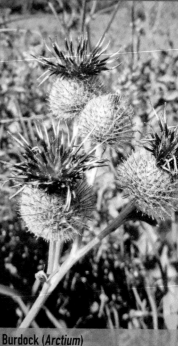

Black Raspberry (*Rubus occidentalis*)
Carminative, antispasmodic, antidiuretic, astringent

Yarrow (*Achillea millefolium*)
Diaphoretic, astringent, tonic, stimulant

White Oak (*Quercus alba*)
Astringent

Burdock (*Arctium*)
Detoxifier

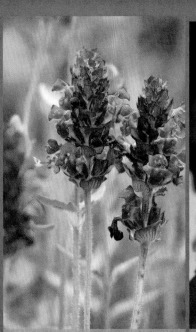

**Heal All, a.k.a. Woundwort
(*Prunella vulgaris*)**
Cooling, antiseptic, immune system balance

Jewelweed (*Impatiens capensis*)
Anti-inflammatory, antihistamine

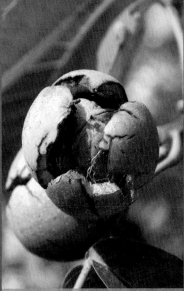

Black Walnut (*Juglans nigra*)
Astringent, antiseptic, vermifuge

Staghorn Sumac (*Rhus typhina*)
Cooling, antiseptic, astringent, styptic

7

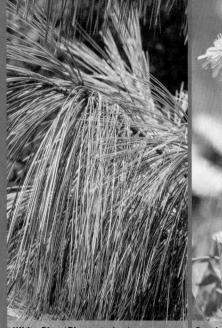

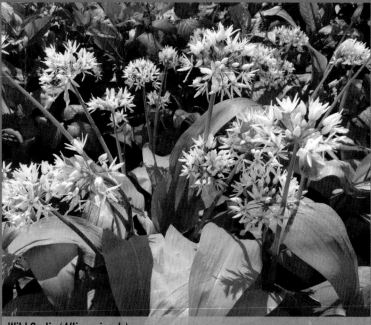

White Pine (*Pinus strobus*)
Antibacterial, antifungal

Dandelion (*Taraxacum officinale*)
Diuretic, anti-inflammatory, tonic

Wild Garlic (*Allium vineale*)
Antiasthmatic, carminative, diuretic, expectorant, hypotensive, stimulant, vasodilator

HONEYSUCKLE (*Lonicera*)

Taste: Sweet

Areas found: Often invasive and climbing among trees and low shrubs in areas at the edge of fields and older roads

Description: There are around twenty types of honeysuckle in North America. Whether it is the shrub or the climbing-vine variety, honeysuckle is easily recognized by its fragrant, trumpet-shaped flowers, which bloom in an array of colors, from white to yellow to red. When not in bloom honeysuckle bears bright-colored berries that attract various birds.

Medicinal actions: Antibacterial, anti-inflammatory, antispasmodic, diuretic, fever reducer

Uses: A decoction of honeysuckle stems is used internally in the treatment of acute rheumatoid arthritis, mumps, and hepatitis. Honeysuckle stems and flowers are used together as a medicinal infusion in the treatment of upper respiratory tract infections (including pneumonia) and dysentery. It can be used internally and externally to treat any inflammation.

See insert, page 5

BLACK CHERRY (*Prunus serotina*)

Taste: Bitter, sweet, sour

Areas found: Hardwood areas of the Eastern Woodlands

Description: Fairly large tree with bark that peels and is red underneath. The outer bark is usually a dark gray.

Medicinal actions: Astringent

Uses: The root bark and inner bark can be used in infusions (not boiled) to treat diarrhea, fever, coughs, colds, and sore throats.

See insert, page 5

WOOD SORREL (*Oxalis stricta*)

Taste: Cooling, sour

Areas found: Field edges

Description: Leaves are clover-like with yellow flowers.

Medicinal actions: Cooling, tonic, anti-inflammatory

Uses: Decoctions are used to relieve hemorrhages and urinary disorders. Cloths soaked with juice and applied to the skin are effective in the reduction of swellings and inflammation. Don't overuse wood sorrel internally.

Other plants for hot tissue states:

- Hawthorn
- Sheep sorrel
- Garden sorrel
- Lavender

See insert, page 5

PLANTS FOR
WET CONDITIONS

BLACK RASPBERRY (*Rubus occidentalis*)

Taste: Fruit is sweet, tart, sour; leaves a bit less but still citrus

Areas found: Eastern Woodlands

Description: A very common woodland plant, it grows in thickets and is covered in thorns. The fruit can be bright red to almost black depending on ripeness, and the leaves are generally in clusters of three at the end of each branch. This plant, like many others, will most often be found on edges of fields and clearings.

Medicinal actions: Carminative, antispasmodic, antidiuretic, astringent

Uses: Alleviates menstrual cramps, diarrhea, colds, and stomach complaints. Raspberry tea can reduce fever.

See insert, page 6

YARROW (*Achillea millefolium*)

Taste: Astringent

Areas found: Everywhere, along roadways, paths, meadows, pastures

Description: It blooms from June to September. This plant is fairly easily identified in the summer when blooming as it has a white flower top with many small flowers, creating a doily-looking flower head. The leaves are similar to fine feathers. However, it can be confused with Queen Anne's lace and hemlock so correct identification is imperative with this species. This is one of the most-used plants due to its blood-clotting capabilities as well as work on fevers.

Medicinal actions: Diaphoretic (a substance that induces sweating), astringent, tonic, stimulant, and mild aromatic

Uses: It can be used to treat deep lacerations, bleeding, severe colds, and flu. It induces perspiration and is a mild stimulant.

See insert, page 6

WHITE OAK (*Quercus alba*)

Taste: Acorns can be sweet

Areas found: Common in eastern and central North America

Description: White oak leaves lack the points on the lobes that are indicative of a red oak species. You can also cut into the cambium layer of bark and it will be white or red.

Medicinal actions: Astringent

Uses: The ground bark or the meat from an acorn is heavily astringent for minor bleeding, but the white oak has been traditionally used for any wet tissue state externally as well as internally from the neck up or within the digestive tract.

See insert, page 6

BURDOCK (*Arctium*)

Taste: Dry

Areas found: Near older homesteads, and roadsides, especially many back roads; disturbed soil

Description: Large-leaf plant that can be mistaken for rhubarb. Identify by the spike in the center with many attached burrs in the stem.

Medicinal actions: Traditionally used to clear toxins from the bloodstream

Uses: Used externally, it can relieve skin problems such as eczema, acne, and psoriasis. Taken internally, it helps eliminate excess water. Pregnant or nursing women should not take burdock.

See insert, page 6

HEAL ALL, A.K.A. WOUNDWORT
(*Prunella vulgaris*)

Taste: Dry

Areas found: Open field edges and open fields, sometimes near thickets

Description: Smaller plant that grows in clusters, it has few leaves but a longer squarish stem. Top resembles a cone with many small blue-purple flowers in season.

Medicinal actions: Cooling, antiseptic, immune system balance

Uses: Externally, used for healing wounds and sores. Internally, used to relieve eye inflammation and eyestrain, to treat digestive tract problems, and to relieve headaches and sore throats.

See insert, page 7

JEWELWEED (*Impatiens capensis*)

Taste: Not edible

Areas found: Wet drainages and creek beds

Description: Grows in large patches, has a hollow stem that contains some liquid. Nodules grow at each intersection; flowers are orange when blooming.

Medicinal actions: Anti-inflammatory, antihistamine

Uses: Jewelweed contains a compound called lawsone in its leaves, which has been proven to have antihistamine and anti-inflammatory properties when used as a salve.

See insert, page 7

BLACK WALNUT (*Juglans nigra*)

Taste: Acrid

Areas found: Wood lines within fields and along roadways, especially in old settled areas

Description: Large tree generally appears in poor health in the winter months. Heavily furrowed bark, many lance-shaped leaves. Pith of stem and tree are brown, and it bears a green-hulled nut in season.

Medicinal actions: Astringent, antiseptic, vermifuge (for treating intestinal parasites)

Uses: It oxygenates the blood, killing parasites. It can balance sugar levels and burn up excessive toxins and fatty materials. The juice from the fruit husk is applied externally as a treatment for ringworm. An infusion of the bark can be used to treat diarrhea.

See insert, page 7

STAGHORN SUMAC (*Rhus typhina*)

Taste: Tart

Areas found: Throughout the Eastern Woodlands especially in wood lines near clearing and disturbed agricultural areas

Description: A smaller tree, it bears a red fruit in a large cluster during bloom. The bark has a milky sap when cut.

Medicinal actions: Cooling, antiseptic, astringent, styptic

Uses: An infusion of sumac bark or roots is antiseptic, astringent, and diuretic. It is used for the treatment of colds, diarrhea, fevers, general debility, to increase the flow of breast milk, to treat sore mouths and throats, rectal bleeding, inflammation of the bladder and painful urination, retention of urine and dysentery, and is applied externally to treat excessive vaginal discharge, burns, and skin eruptions.

See insert, page 7

WHITE PINE (*Pinus strobus*)

Taste: Pungent, warm

Areas found: Throughout the Eastern Woodlands in sandy soils

Description: The easiest way to identify white pine is by its clusters of five needles.

Medicinal actions: Antibacterial, antifungal

Uses: Of all the trees that produce medicine, perhaps the most versatile is the white pine. Nearly every part of it serves a medicinal purpose. The needles, which can be easily made into an herbal tea, provide high amounts of vitamin C to strengthen the immune system. The sap, frequently referred to as pitch or resin, is both antibacterial and antifungal; it also works well to stop bleeding, seal wounds, and draw out things that shouldn't be there such as pus or splinters. The inner bark contains natural oils and resins that have antiseptic and expectorant qualities. *Note*: Avoid infusions of long-needled pine species.

See insert, page 8

DANDELION (*Taraxacum officinale*)

Taste: Bitter

Areas found: Open fields, and beaten pathways, in full sun generally, common yard plant

Description: Wide green leaves in a ground rosette; sometimes also grows in clusters; long hollow stem with yellow flower in season.

Medicinal actions: Diuretic, anti-inflammatory, tonic

Uses: Dandelion is used to treat kidney and urinary disorders and as a diuretic. It can also be used for eczema and acne.

See insert, page 8

WILD GARLIC (*Allium vineale*)

Taste: Aromatic, pungent

Areas found: Fields especially in agricultural areas, and woodland edges

Description: Similar to an onion with a multiple-lobed bulb underground and thin, long green stems above with a white flower in season.

Medicinal actions: Antiasthmatic, carminative, diuretic, expectorant, hypotensive, stimulant, and vasodilator

Uses: The raw root can be eaten to reduce blood pressure and also to ease shortness of breath.

Other medicinal plants for wet conditions:

- Chickweed

> **BUSHCRAFT TIP**
> Honey is a versatile natural substance that can help treat many common problems from minor burns to skin wounds to infections. Keep raw honey on hand for quick and handy first aid (plus it tastes great on campfire biscuits!).

See insert, page 8

OPOSSUM MENTALITY REGARDING MEDICINAL PLANTS

In the Pathfinder System, there is a concept we refer to as "Opossum Mentality," which means, when you see it grab it for later use. In a wilderness emergency situation, the best herb you can have is the one you have at hand. The more you learn to identify medicinal plants, the better prepared you will be to pick them up as you walk around in the wild. The more varieties you pick, the more treatment options you will have should you need to rely on their medicinal properties. So, train yourself to pick up medicinal herbs and wild foods as you see them just as you would collect fire-making materials for the next fire.

PROCESSING HERBS FOR MEDICINAL USE

Herbs can be prepared in different ways to fully access their various healing properties. Here are some of the most common methods of processing herbs.

Poultice: Ground, masticated, or shredded herbs usually moistened and packed over the skin and then wrapped to keep in place. Poultices are used to relieve soreness and inflammation.

Hot infusion: An infusion uses water, oil, or alcohol to extract chemical compounds from plants. For a hot infusion, use hot solvents. Generally the water (or oil or alcohol) is heated and poured over the plant material, then left to steep for about fifteen minutes. (Decoctions are used for roots and barks, infusions for leaves and flowering tops.)

Cold infusion: Cold infusions are used for herbs that lose their effectiveness when exposed to heat, such as peppermint, sumac, lemon, and lemon balm. Cold infusions are used to gain a cooling action. Cold (even frozen) solvents are used.

Decoction: For harder-to-extract herbs such as roots and bark, decoction is used to concentrate the active ingredient of a plant by heating or boiling it.

Tincture: An herb preserved in liquid, generally vodka/brandy or glycerin.

Fomentations: Cloth dipped in a decoction or infusion and applied to the skin.

Salves: The mixture of an oil with the herb plus beeswax. These are used for topical/external applications and can protect the skin while helping to heal a wound.

Crushed application: Some herbs can be used straight from the plant with little preparation beyond crushing them to release their juices.

PREPARING A FRESH-HERB POULTICE

If using fresh herbs for your poultice, place 2 ounces of chopped or bruised herbs—about ½ cup—and a cup of water in a small saucepan. Simmer for 2 minutes. Do not drain. Arrange a clean piece of gauze, muslin, linen, or white cotton sheet on a clean, flat surface. The material should be large enough to cover the affected area completely (but do not place on the affected area yet). Remove the hot herbs from the saucepan. When cool enough to be placed on skin and not scald, place the hot herbs directly on the skin you are treating. Then pour the herbal solution over the cloth and place the cloth over the herbs that are on the skin. Wrap a towel around the poultice to prevent the soiling of clothes.

Hot poultices are best for superficial wounds. The heat helps to draw blood to the surface, opens the pores, and assists in the assimilation of the herbs through the skin. This is great for wet and unproductive coughs.

Cold poultices are best for deep wounds, such as contusions, bruises, and fractures. The affected area will usually feel hot to touch and so the cold poultice (made either by preparing herbs with cold water, or by cooling a previously prepared one) will act as an analgesic, helping to draw the beneficial effects of the herbs down deep into the tissue.

Herbal poultices should be kept in place for one to twenty-four hours, or as needed. During this period, you may experience a throbbing pain as the poultice draws out infection and neutralizes toxins. When the pain subsides, you will know that the poultice has accomplished its task and should be removed. Apply fresh poultices as needed until the desired level of healing has been reached.

HOT INFUSION (HOT TEA)

1. Shred 8 ounces fresh herbs (4 ounces dried) and place in pitcher or bowl. Boil 1 quart water in bush pot. Pour the boiling water over the fresh shredded herbs.
2. Cover the brew and remove from the heat.
3. Let it steep for 5–15 minutes. Generally an infusion made from roots or bark should be left to steep longer than those made from flowers or leaves. If fresh plants are used, it tends to infuse much faster compared to dried plants.
4. After steeping the herbal tea for the appropriate amount of time, filter out the liquid. Drink 8 ounces every 1–2 hours until gone.

DECOCTION

1. Pour the required amount of water into a container and bring the water to a boil. Generally use about 1 cup of water.

2. Add in the required amount of the plant parts. Use 2–4 tablespoons of fresh herbs. Continue simmering over low heat for 15–30 minutes.
3. Remove from heat and let the brew stand for a few minutes.
4. Strain the liquid out while it is still hot. Drink 8 ounces every 1–2 hours.

COLD INFUSION

Cold infusions are made like a sun tea, with cold water poured over the herb and then left in the sun to steep. They take longer than hot infusions to pull the good stuff from the plant matter but also have certain advantages in cases where heat could damage some of the constituents of the plant.

TINCTURE

Tinctures, although not practical for on-the-trail preparations, are an inexpensive and potent way to preserve and use medicinal herbs. Although the quantities of vodka/brandy vary, most herbal tinctures are very easy to make and will last for years at full potency. If you desire to use wild picked or store-bought dried herbs for your family's health needs, tincturing is worth learning as it will provide you inexpensive, fast-acting remedies with less work than tea.

A simple alcohol tincture is made by using at least 90 proof liquor of any kind. Stuff a dark bottle or jar with plant materials, then add liquor to the top and seal. Store in a dark place for approximately two weeks, shaking the contents every day for the first week. Then strain and use in drops as a medicinal preparation.

FOMENTATIONS

Dip a cloth or towel in a warm infusion or decoction, wring it out, and apply locally to the affected body part. Cover the cloth with a dry towel to help retain the heat. These herbal preparations are used to treat headaches, chest congestion, skin irritations, and swelling due to an injury. They can be used hot or cold. Use cold compresses where the skin is broken or feels flushed. Use hot compresses when the skin is not broken and/or circulation needs to be brought to the area.

As with herbal poultices, fomentations should be kept in place for one to twenty-four hours, or as needed, and again, you may experience a throbbing pain as the fomentation draws out infection and neutralizes toxins. When the pain subsides, you will know that the fomentation has accomplished its task and should be removed. Apply fresh fomentations as needed until the desired level of healing has been reached.

SALVES

Salves can be made in many ways, but the simplest method is to use a combination of olive oil or another carrier oil and beeswax. Then add the herb and let simmer for about 20 minutes. A simple way to check the consistency is to spoon out a bit of liquid and allow it to cool. It should be solid but creamy, like petroleum jelly. You can make the salve wetter or dryer, according to your personal preference, by adjusting the amount of oil and beeswax you use and by adjusting the simmer time. When satisfied with the consistency, remove it from the heat and let cool. Store in a tin or small, wide-mouthed glass container.

COMMON CONDITIONS AND THEIR TREATMENTS	
CONDITION	TREATMENT
Bleeding	White oak bark (poultice); black walnut (powder)
Breaks, sprains, strains	White oak (fomentation, cool)
Bites, stings	Charcoal poultice (must be kept warm)

COMMON CONDITIONS AND THEIR TREATMENTS

CONDITION	TREATMENT
Blisters	Plantain salve
Burns	Honey; plantain salve (do not use either on severe burns)
Constipation	Black walnut (mild decoction)
Diarrhea	White oak (strong decoction); white or black willow (strong decoction); black walnut (mild decoction)
Stomach upset (possible poison)	Charcoal (purgative: mix 1 teaspoon with 4 ounces water)
Stomach upset (gas, cramps, indigestion)	Charcoal (½ teaspoon with 12 ounces water)
Immune system	Honey (1 teaspoon 3 times per day)
Sore throat	White oak bark (mild decoction); black walnut (mild decoction)
Cough	White oak bark (strong decoction)
Sleeplessness	White or black willow (strong decoction)
Headache	White or black willow (mild decoction)
Fever	White or black willow bark (strong decoction)
Minor abrasions	Honey (use as ointment); plantain salve
Toothache, mouth sores	Honey; white oak bark (strong decoction); sea salt (1 teaspoon per 4 ounces water; use as mouthwash)
PMS	Willow (decoction)
UTI	White oak (mild decoction); black walnut (strong decoction)
Antiparasitic (bad water)	Black walnut (strong decoction: 50/50 leaves/hulls, if possible)
Fight or flight	White or black willow (mild decoction)
Contact dermatitis	Black walnut (mild decoction, fomentation); charcoal (poultice on irruptions)
Electrolytes imbalance	Honey and sea salt (1 teaspoon honey and ⅛ teaspoon sea salt dissolved in 8 ounces water)

TIPS AND TRICKS

- Remember that most plants that are medicine are also food, or at least edible, so if you don't have time for a preparation to be taken internally, just eat the plant.
- A spit poultice is a quick way to use a topical medicinal. Just chew the plant and mix with saliva, then pack over the affected area and bandage.
- An infusion can always be used as a wash to help speed healing.

— Appendix 1 —
LEGAL AND ETHICAL CONSIDERATIONS

The most important task of rescuers is to rescue. What you've learned in this book are techniques that will help injured people in the wild (as well as you) and quite possibly save lives. That said, things don't always go according to the book. When helping an injured person, you may commit a mistake, possibly even one that does additional harm. Unfortunately, in today's litigious society, you may get sued.

What should you do? The easiest thing would be to back off and offer no help. But this would be profoundly wrong. Your first instinct, to help the injured or ill person, is the right one. Be aware that each state has different laws regarding the administration of first aid and what legal obligations you may have.

The Wilderness Medical Society has developed a set of legal principles for emergency care to help you decide what to do. In general, legally you don't have to help a stranger unless you have a business relationship with him or are in a position where it is expected that you will give aid. For example, a park ranger would be expected to render first aid. So, too, would a wilderness group leader if someone in the party is hurt. When the injured person is not a stranger or if you helped create the dangerous situation, you are generally expected to give aid. For example, a parent would be expected to help his child. If you accidentally drove your ATV over someone's foot, you'd be expected to help as well.

No one expects you to have the same level of first-aid skills as a medical professional; if you feel that a situation is beyond your abilities, work to evacuate the patient as quickly as possible so that he can receive professional assistance. Never accept money in return for care, as this violates most Good Samaritan laws designed to protect aid givers.

In many situations, the factor that caused the injury continues to endanger all those in the area. You should never put the health and safety of the victim above your own. However, once you've begun to help someone, you must remain there until relieved by someone with the same or greater level of first-aid skills. If helping an injured or ill person would risk your own life or safety, you are not expected to help.

If the injured person is alert, treat him as a partner in his own care. Ask if it's okay for you to help. Be calm, rational, and if he objects, tell him why what you're suggesting is the best course. If he's confused (which, depending on the injury, he may well be) or could hurt himself further by his actions, you're permitted to help. If the injured person is unresponsive, it is assumed that he would consent to treatment and so you may act.

Since you want to gain his confidence, start by explaining who you are and how much training you've had in first aid. Always tell him why you're doing what you're doing ("I'm splinting your leg to immobilize it until we can get you to a doctor").

In short, the law doesn't compel you to help someone who's ill or injured in the wilderness. But if you're a good person, and we assume you are, you'll feel obliged to use what you've learned from this book to help.

— Appendix 2 —

CREATING FIRST-AID KITS

If you're planning a wilderness trip, you may want to devise a first-aid kit for use in the event of an accident or illness. The tools and supplies can be customized for your needs—for example, a first-aid kit can be designed for self-aid or for group camp use. Requirements will differ depending on group size, trip length, remoteness of location, and your individual or group medical qualifications, but these should serve as a solid foundation from which to build.

SELF-AID KIT

Generally, we rely heavily on the Ten Cs as the basis for improvised self-aid supplemented by simple over-the-counter pain relievers and herbal medicines and medicinal salves. Thus, our recommended self-aid kit would include:

- ❏ Cutting tools (knife, axe, saw)
- ❏ Combustion devices (fire-starting tools)
- ❏ Cover elements (clothing, tarps, tents)
- ❏ Cordage (bank line and paracord)

- ❑ Containers (32-ounce stainless steel bottle at minimum)
- ❑ Compass (with mirror and built-in magnification lens)
- ❑ Cargo tape (Gorilla Tape)
- ❑ Candling device (headlamp with spare batteries)
- ❑ Cloth (3' × 3' of cotton cloth)
- ❑ Canvas needle (for equipment repairs)
- ❑ Woodsman's apothecary
  - ❑ Acetaminophen
  - ❑ Ibuprofen
  - ❑ Diphenhydramine (antihistamine)
  - ❑ Camp wax
  - ❑ Nitrile gloves

BUSHCRAFT TIP

If firearms will be involved in your trip, consider including a tactical first-aid kit:

- ❑ Tourniquets
- ❑ Chest seals
- ❑ Duct tape
- ❑ Nitrile gloves
- ❑ Quick clot
- ❑ Steri-Strips
- ❑ Dermabond or Vetbond

BASE CAMP FIRST-AID KIT

This kit design is for the needs of multiple people within the same group. Trained responders may wish to substitute elements to better suit their needs according to their level of training.

- ❑ Protect any sterile dressings within your kit from moisture by sealing them in 1-gallon freezer bags in groups of four.
- ❑ Your kit should always be easily accessible and its location known by everyone in your group.

❑ A designated person, typically the one with the most training, should be appointed medical person in charge.

❑ Label all containers clearly and include instructions in case the medical person in charge is the one who becomes injured.

❑ Splints can be improvised in the field from natural material or foam sleeping pads. So only include SAM splints if you have space or the desire to carry them.

BANDAGES AND DRESSINGS

❑ 4" × 4" gauze pads
❑ 2" × 2" gauze pads
❑ 3" gauze roller bandage
❑ Paper tape
❑ Elastic roller bandage
❑ Self-adhering bandage
❑ Cravat
❑ Adhesive bandages (various sizes)
❑ Steri-Strips or butterfly bandages
❑ Wound irrigation syringe
❑ 1½" athletic tape
❑ 2nd Skin
❑ Moleskin

OINTMENTS AND MEDICATIONS

❑ Povidone iodine
❑ Triple antibiotic cream
❑ Cortizone cream
❑ Aspirin
❑ Ibuprofen
❑ Acetaminophen
❑ Diphenhydramine (antihistamine)
❑ Hydration salts/Jell-O

TOOLS

- ❑ Bandage scissors/EMT shears
- ❑ Thermometer with hard case
- ❑ Tweezers
- ❑ Nitrile gloves
- ❑ Sawyer Extractor
- ❑ Notepad and pencil
- ❑ Small multitool or Swiss Army knife
- ❑ Emergency space blanket
- ❑ Safety glasses and face shield

AIRWAY DEVICES

- ❑ CPR mask
- ❑ Nasopharyngeal airway

SIGNAL DEVICES

- ❑ Signal mirror
- ❑ Road flare
- ❑ Headlamp and batteries

INDEX